"Finally, a lunch book with a focus on health! Laura knows how to take the panic out of making daily lunch and serves up ideas parents can actually manage. This book should be required reading!"

—MELISSA LANZ, author of *The Fresh 20 Cookbook*

"Variety, lunch-packing tips, and food pictured how it's actually sent to school—this book takes the guesswork out of how to pack fresh lunches your kids will love."

—KELLY LESTER, founder of EasyLunchboxes.com

"*The Best Homemade Kids' Lunches on the Planet* is an invaluable resource for any busy parent who struggles with the day-to-day task of packing a healthy lunch. It is filled with strategies for shopping, delicious food combinations, and creative lunches with whole-food ingredients."

—AMY CLARK, founder of MomAdvice.com

"Laura Fuentes' emphasis on real, fresh, kid-pleasing food gives parents plenty of healthy combinations for picky eaters. I also like the battle-tested tips for fighting soggy bread!"

—HEATHER GIBBS FLETT, co-author of *The Rookie Mom's Handbook* and *Stuff Every Mom Should Know*

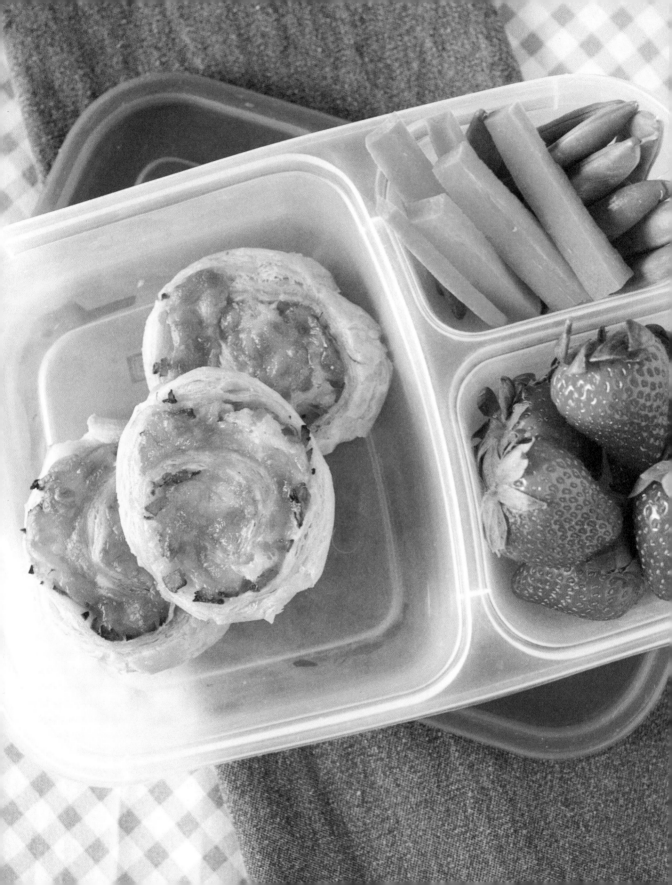

THE BEST HOMEMADE KIDS' LUNCHES ON THE PLANET

Make Lunches Your kids Will Love
with More Than 200 Deliciously Nutritious
Meal Ideas

Laura Fuentes
Founder of MOMables.com

Fair Winds Press
100 Cummings Center, Suite 406L
Beverly, MA 01915

fairwindspress.com • quarryspoon.com

© 2014 Fair Winds Press

First published in the USA in 2014 by
Fair Winds Press, a member of
Quarto Publishing Group USA Inc.
100 Cummings Center
Suite 406-L
Beverly, MA 01915-6101
www.fairwindspress.com
Visit www.QuarrySPOON.com and help us celebrate food and culture one spoonful at a time!

18 17 16 15 14   5

ISBN: 978-1-59233-608-1

Digital edition published in 2014
eISBN: 978-1-62788-025-1

Library of Congress Cataloging-in-Publication Data available

Cover and book design by Carol Holtz
Page layout: *tabula rasa* graphic design
Photography by Alison Bickel Photography
Printed and bound in Canada

The information in this book is for educational purposes only. It is not intended to replace the advice of a physician or medical practitioner. Please see your health care provider before beginning any new health program.

For my Abuela, who inspired my love for fresh food—
I will always feel your presence in my kitchen.

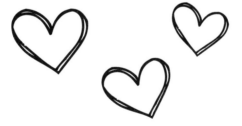

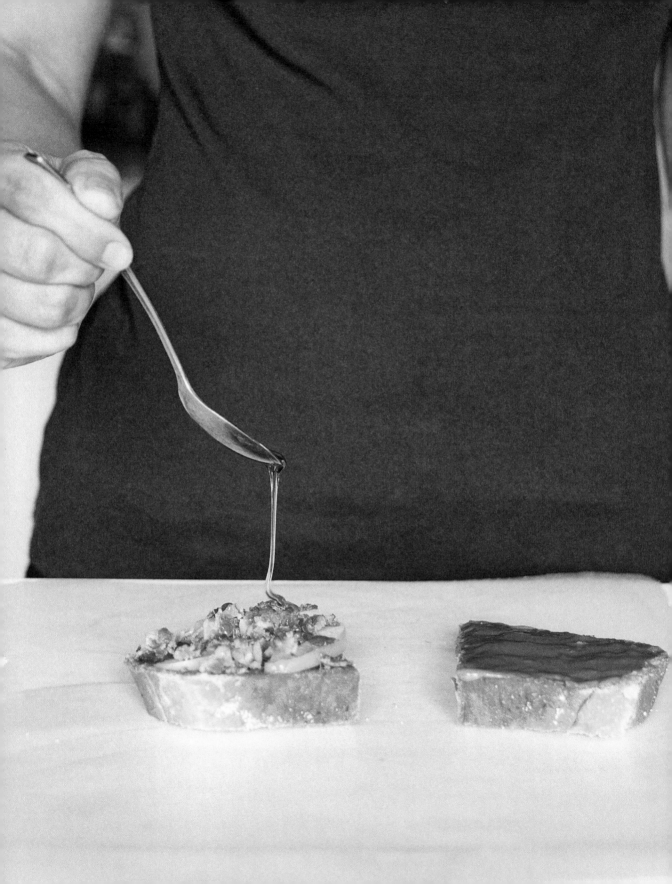

CONTENTS

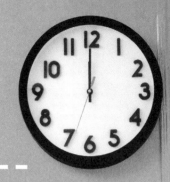

INTRODUCTION

I used to stare at the refrigerator every morning, waiting for food to talk to me and say, "Pick me! Pack me inside the lunchbox!" Unfortunately, the longer I stared, the longer the food stayed silent.

At the grocery store, I swear those brightly colored boxes holding premade lunches would actually speak to my daughter, saying "I am fun! You'll love me for lunch! And don't tell your mom, but I have really bad ingredients!"

I remember the first week of my daughter's two-day-a-week preschool. I was so excited to make perfect little lunches with fresh fruits and neatly stacked veggies. I also remember the disappointment I felt three weeks later when I didn't know what else to pack for her. The truth: I was stumped for ideas.

Adding to my lack of ideas were food allergies to take into consideration. After extensive food journaling, I was able to determine that my little girl was allergic to disodium phosphates and chemical nitrates. Fortunately, the easiest way to avoid these is to purchase real foods, including natural and organic meats, and become food label savvy.

But at that point in my life, I had a two-month-old at home, I was sleep-deprived, and time was of the essence. While I could cook just about anything, I wasn't very organized in the kitchen (yet), so we were spending more money than I would have liked for healthy convenience foods—and I was becoming a short-order cook.

By the time my oldest kids were two and three years old, they were both attending preschool a few days a week. Because they didn't complain about the same lunches being served often, I continued to do the same rotation of three lunches for them. Yet, inside, I knew I could and should do better.

One day, I ran out of sandwich bread, and I decided to use leftover pancakes from breakfast night instead. That lunch was immediately a hit with my daughter, and her excitement and request for more fun lunches was all the motivation I needed to do better.

From that day forward, and for the past four years, I've been giving kid-appeal to real foods, making my own versions of those store-bought lunches that kids like so much with fresh ingredients, and helping thousands feed their children better school lunches through MOMables.com.

Along the way, I've learned how to pack foods so that they don't become soggy inside the lunchbox, tested nearly every lunch container out there, and developed hundreds of recipes.

I attribute much of my creativity to my two oldest kids being very picky eaters. They often refuse to try new foods and continue to be a challenge in the kitchen. Most of the recipes I develop are my attempts at sneaking more nutrition into foods my oldest two will actually eat. My youngest, on the other hand, is the complete opposite. He was born six months after I launched MOMables and, since then, has volunteered much of his time to taste-testing many of my recipes. Thankfully, he is nearly always willing to try something new!

This book has many of my family's favorite recipes and kitchen shortcuts, so you can make lunches quickly and healthfully. I also share my tips on how to freeze, store, and repurpose leftovers, so that less food is wasted and you can stretch your grocery budget even further.

Not only that, but you'll also be able to use the recipes whether you have kids in kinder-garten or high school, because the recipes in this book can be adjusted for portion size. And, if you really want to go all out in lunch packing, you can be like my family and use these recipes for adults too. They're made for everyone!

Packing a healthy school lunch should not be complicated. All you need are some great recipes, fresh ingredients, and the willingness to try a few new things. I hope that in the following pages, you find inspiration to make lunchtime a success!

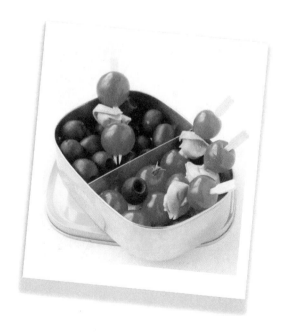

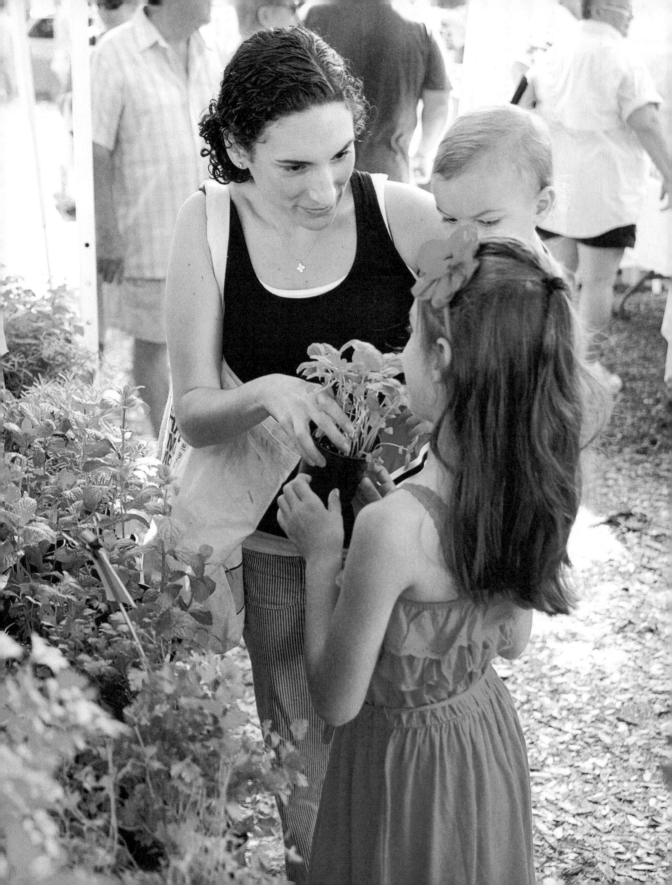

CHAPTER 1

PACK LIKE A PRO: NOURISHING FOODS ON THE GO

In this chapter, I'll walk you through everything you need to know to get started with packing the best lunches possible for everyone in your family. From budget-friendly shopping tips to smart strategies for packing and creating healthful meals, it's all covered here!

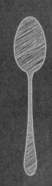

Shopping: Real Food for Busy Families

Fresh is best. That's what my grandmother used to say. Whether you go to the grocery store once a month, once a week, or even once a day, you should purchase the freshest, most wholesome ingredients your budget can afford.

If you have a farmers' market, check out what's offered there, and use that as a guide to what you should be buying fresh, even at the grocery. The least expensive produce is always the one *in season* and not the kind that is imported from remote parts of the globe.

I wish I could say that I have access to everything organic and that I do all my grocery shopping in one stop, but I can't. Unfortunately, I don't have a huge organic grocery section near me, a well-stocked farmers' market, or a great selection of trusted brands at my favorite supermarket. Because of this, I pick and choose where I purchase certain supplies. I have a routine and a list of the groceries that I buy at each of my three stops. In addition, I purchase some items online in bulk at lower prices.

I've become savvy about feeding my family fresh food while staying within our budget. The single most important thing that has helped me get creative with our meals at an affordable price is meal planning.

How do I do it? It's a lot easier than you might think! To start, I spend ten to twenty minutes each Saturday or Sunday looking at recipes, bookmarking those I want to make, writing down the ingredients I'll need, and creating a shopping list. After that, I head out to my stops with my list and a big iced coffee, to purchase the freshest food I can find.

I then spend most of my Sunday around the kitchen, cooking a big family meal for that evening and prepping for the week ahead. While my children are young (seven, six, and twenty-one months), they are beginning to help with easy tasks, such as washing produce and putting things away, and often help me cook simple things. My seven-year-old daughter has mastered the toaster oven, so getting them involved, even in the simplest of tasks, has been instrumental to pulling this all off. I am convinced that if I can do it, so can you!

Try meal planning for a week or two, and see what you think. Once it's part of your routine, it should make life easier for you! And if you need a little help, check out the sample plans at the end of this book, which should help inspire you!

HOMEMADE VERSUS STORE-BOUGHT

Before I had kids, I used to see those packaged lunches at the grocery store and think "Wow! A whole meal for a couple of bucks? That's crazy cheap!" I now know *cheap* is the key word there. Those meals have cheap foods, poor nutritional content, and unidentifiable ingredients—quick and convenient, perhaps, but not something I'd want to give my children.

Instead, I purchase organic meats without chemical nitrates and preservatives, organic or antibiotic-free cheese, and organic produce whenever possible. I make my own treats and use reusable lunch containers. I've done the math, and the numbers don't lie; my homemade, organic version of the convenient, store-bought lunch is still cheaper!

I used to think that *all* organic food was more expensive. My perception of buying organic was that it was only for those wealthy enough, and those who couldn't afford it had to settle for less expensive (read: lower-quality) ingredients. But when I had my first child and got serious about wholesome eating, I discovered that I was often loading my grocery cart with organic convenience items that I didn't need and therefore spending a lot more than I should. Organic basics, on the other hand, such as meat and produce, could more easily fit into my budget and be turned into great, affordable meals. By sticking with a weekly plan for my food, I can stretch my food budget and afford to purchase certain ingredients organic, hormone-free, free range, unprocessed— you know, the ones that I thought would cause me to go over budget way back then.

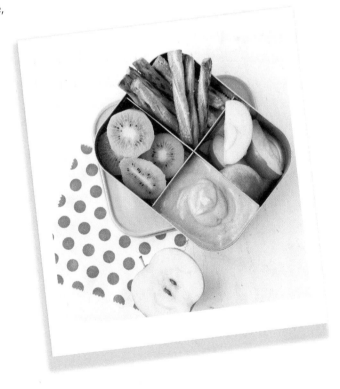

FRESH FOOD DOESN'T HAVE TO BREAK THE BANK

When I sat down to write this book, I wanted to make sure the recipes here went beyond the sandwich and that you also got many of my homemade staples (such as pesto, jams, and hummus), which are much cheaper to make at home and often better tasting! There are a few other easy ways to save money when packing your own lunches as well.

The first is choosing foods that are inexpensive by nature, such as pasta, rice, eggs, potatoes, and whole grains. These items will build the bulk of your meal, so you'll be providing nutrition while not spending a lot of money. Meat, especially organic, can be expensive, so by not making it the main focus of your lunchbox, you'll be able to stretch your dollar further (and it's easy to get protein in other ways).

Second, when certain fruits and vegetables are not in season, buying them frozen can be a lot more cost effective. I prefer frozen vegetables to canned, because they were flash frozen at their ripest and juiciest for maximum flavor, and have nothing added.

Budget-Friendly Lunchbox Foods

The following are my top cheap-and-healthy items for lunchboxes and beyond:

- Apples
- Bananas
- Berries (in season)
- Bulk beans
- Homemade breads
- Rice
- Whole grain pasta
- Eggs
- Frozen fruits and veggies
- Carrots
- Nut butters

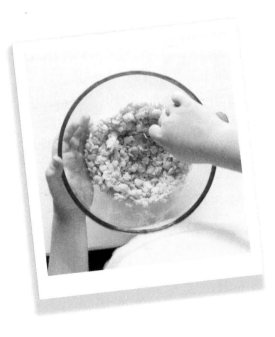

Stocking Your Fridge, Freezer, and Pantry

I used to think that making my own lunches would take a lot of time and require many ingredients. But one day, I took a closer look at the foods that were in our daily meal rotation, and it hit me: Most of the meals we were eating shared the same basic ingredients! For lunch prep, I could easily use some of the dinner ingredients and repurpose them in creative ways!

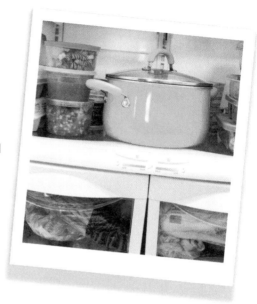

From that day on, I began to stock my pantry with items that would not only go far and stretch our budget but also allow me to make my family's favorite foods and treats from scratch—quickly and easily.

The fridge, freezer, and pantry basics you'll find listed here are the basis of most of the recipes in this book. They are the staples I keep on hand at almost all times, because they can be easily mixed-and-matched to create a wide array of recipes. Use these lists as a guide, purchasing those items you think you'll get the most use out of or already have bookmarked as part of your recipe and menu planning. The brand and variety of products you choose to purchase will of course depend on your family's preferences and needs.

STOCKING YOUR FRIDGE

Because dairy items such as cheese, butter, and eggs have a longer shelf life than meats and seafood—and get used up rather quickly—I generally keep these items on hand at all times. Fresh meats and seafood I buy as needed or not more than a few days in advance (unless I plan on freezing them). While research has yet to prove an adverse effect from nonorganic meat consumption, choosing organic meats is a personal choice for us. In addition to taste preference, we purchase organic deli meats to avoid a possible allergic reaction from my daughter. I also like to purchase organic dairy so that it's free from hormones, pesticides, and GMOs (genetically modified organisms). Of course, this is a personal preference.

As for fruits and vegetables, I tend to purchase those that are in season where I live. While they aren't always organic or immediately local, they are definitely cheaper.

Dairy
- Milk
- Butter
- Block of real cheese (for slicing and grating)
- Eggs
- Yogurt
- Cream cheese
- Ricotta cheese

Meats and Seafood
- Nitrate-free organic or natural deli meats
- Nitrate-free organic or natural chicken sausage
- Organic poultry
- Organic grass-fed beef
- White fish and salmon

Fruits and Vegetables
- Apples
- Bananas (countertop storage)
- Grapes
- Carrots
- Celery
- Broccoli
- Lettuce
- Tomatoes (countertop storage)
- Avocados
- Peppers
- Potatoes (pantry storage)
- Onions (pantry storage)
- Fresh herbs

STOCKING YOUR FREEZER

Before the birth of my third child, and shortly after launching my company, my husband and I decided to purchase an extra freezer for our family. Oh my goodness! What a difference this little addition has made!

The garage freezer is mostly stocked with my extra soup portions, make-ahead meals, homemade pizza dough, and baked goods. I love having these items on hand so I can pull what I need out to thaw or warm during busy mornings.

Following are some of my favorite freezer staples:

- Frozen vegetables
- Frozen fruit
- Homemade waffles and pancakes
- Homemade pizza dough
- Homemade chicken nuggets
- Frozen smoothies
- Homemade ice cream
- Homemade cookie dough
- Homemade soups
- Homemade tomato-veggie sauce
- Yeast (I purchase yeast in bulk and store in freezer)
- Ground flax

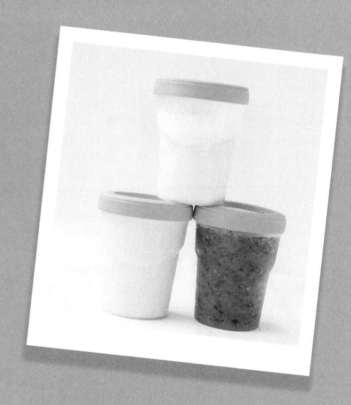

Laura's Tip

Instead of pitching overripe fruit at the end of each week, cut it up and freeze it! Overripe frozen fruit is perfect for smoothies, quick breads, and even our Rainbow Fruit Cups (page 202).

STOCKING YOUR PANTRY

It goes without saying that the smartest way to stock your pantry is with wholesome ingredients you'll actually use! These include whole grains and beans; baking supplies, spices, and sweeteners; and some packaged products.

As I've learned to make many homemade versions of snacks and goodies I used to buy, my packaged-food category has become smaller and smaller over the years. While we used to buy organic cereals for breakfast, for example, we now mostly enjoy homemade baked goods. Lunchbox crackers and treats have also been replaced by many of the recipes you'll find in this book. Broth and stock is usually made from my Sunday roaster chicken, and I make my own pasta sauce so I can sneak in as many veggies as possible. Breads and pizza doughs are also fresh since I purchased my own grain mill and received a bread machine for my birthday one year.

That said, I know most of you want to know how to stock a full pantry—and may not be ready for baking your own bread quite yet!—so I've made the following lists a bit more comprehensive for this reason. Feel free to personalize as best for you and your family.

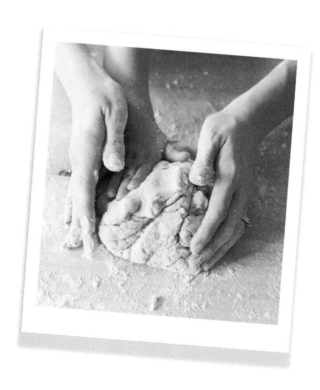

Grains and Legumes

- Rice (brown, white, etc.)
- Pasta
- Quinoa and other bulk grains
- Whole wheat flour
- All-purpose flour
- Oats and oat flour
- Dried beans (red, black, white, chickpeas, lentils)
- Corn kernels for popping

Laura's Tip

To make oat flour, place oats in your food processor or blender and grind until you have a flourlike texture.

Boxed, Canned, and Packaged Goods

- Whole-grain crackers
- Whole wheat bread
- Whole wheat or whole-grain baked goods
- Whole-grain cereals, preferably with no artificial colors and low in sugar
- Canned tomatoes (petite diced or crushed)
- Jarred olives and pickled items
- Condiments

Baking Supplies and Sweeteners

- Sugar
- Honey
- Pure maple syrup
- Baking soda
- Baking powder
- Salt
- Oils (vegetable, extra virgin olive oil, coconut oil)
- Pure vanilla extract
- Vinegar
- Dried fruits
- Nuts
- Ground flaxseed

Spices

- Cinnamon
- Italian seasonings (basil, oregano, rosemary)
- Cumin
- Paprika
- Pepper
- Chili powder
- Garlic powder
- Onion powder
- Parsley
- Dill

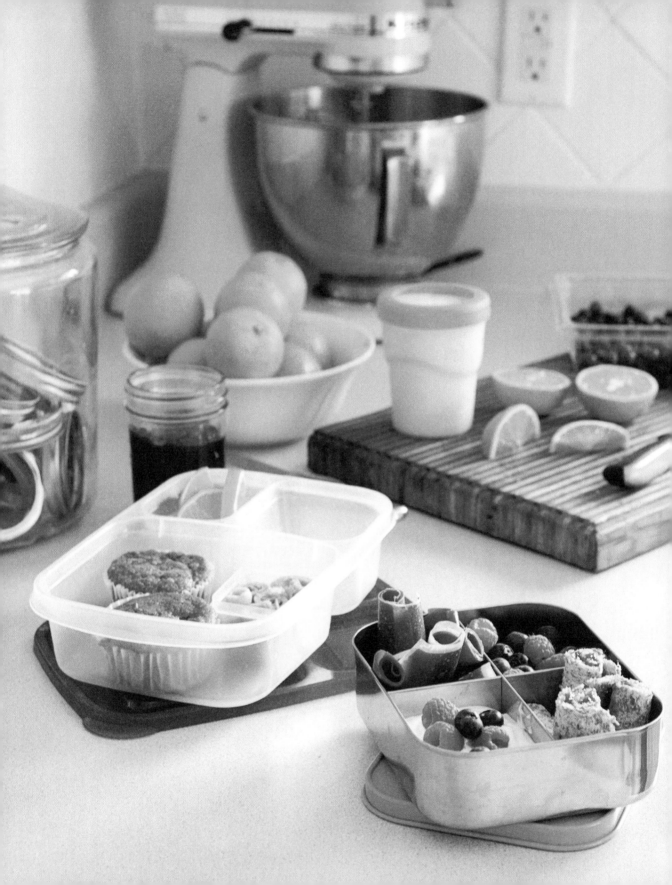

kitchen Gadgets and Lunch Supplies

Myth: You need really cool gadgets, cutters, appliances, and every reusable container out there to make a great lunch.

Truth: All you need are fresh ingredients, something to carry the food in, and the willingness to actually make lunch.

I never ate packed homemade lunches until I moved to the United States (from Spain). In the United States, my mom made my school lunches every morning. Nearly all sandwiches were wrapped in foil; cold pasta salads were sent in old food containers (from yogurt, sour cream, pesto, etc.), and fresh fruit was sent in one piece. She kept it simple. I rarely had the same sandwich twice, however, and loved the feeling of anticipation when I unwrapped my little sandwiches.

Today, we have many different lunch containers available. Many are not worth purchasing, while others I could not live without. They simply make my lunch-packing life easier, and they carry my kids' food without it getting soggy or smashed.

KITCHEN TOOLS

You'll need a cutting board and a good knife to chop fruits and vegetables and put together your sandwiches, a pan or griddle to grill sandwiches and quesadillas, a spatula to flip them, and the patience to stand for a couple of minutes by the stove.

Some of the recipes in this book are family-size meals, so you'll need a pot, a baking dish, and an oven.

A baking pan, bread loaf pan, and cupcake and mini muffin pans are essential to make most of your baked goods and some of the lunch items. The good news is that you can pick up inexpensive ones at many stores near you or online.

LUNCHBOX ESSENTIALS

An insulated lunch bag will shelter homemade lunches and snacks from extreme temperatures. It also protects the food from being squished inside a backpack. The type of lunch bag you purchase will depend on the food containers you like best.

Reusable lunch containers come in all shapes and sizes, plastic or stainless steel, and single compartment or multi-compartment. My favorite lunch containers are those that are affordable, durable, and can be washed in the dishwasher!

If you pack lunches for younger children, make sure they are able to open and close the lunch containers at home prior to sending them to school.

A thermos container is essential if you plan on sending leftovers and warm foods to school. Thermos containers are inexpensive and last a long time; just make sure your child is able to open it at home prior to opening a hot soup at school.

Reusable, inexpensive utensils are also a nice addition to the lunchbox. Ice-packs will help keep the temperature inside the insulated lunch bag cooler longer.

Reusable drink containers are also great to make sure your child has access to fresh water throughout the day. I prefer stainless steel insulated containers because they keep cold water fresh and fresh smoothies cool until lunch.

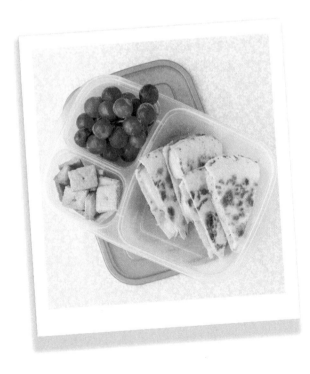

Building the Best Lunchbox for Your Child

What foods should you pack in your child's lunchbox? As a busy parent, it can be difficult to come up with a variety of lunch options that are nutritious, quick to assemble, affordable, and, most important, that your child will actually eat!

When parents join our MOMables community, they often email me seeking ways to add variety to their school lunches, or help with their picky eater, or to find recipes that will make the most of their weekly food budget.

Like them, I am sure most of you are seeking new ideas, too. You want to make things other than the usual peanut butter and jelly sandwich, ham and cheese, and chicken nuggets. You know that nothing is as good as homemade, and you do your best to nourish your child well. And for that, you should be proud!

I must add that the Classroom Cupcakes recipe (page 215) is one you'll never want to live without. Gone are the days where you think a boxed cake mix is the only thing that will yield perfect—and easy—cupcakes for any occasion. Ditch the box and embrace deliciously homemade!

Laura's Tip

Regardless of which lunch containers you choose to purchase, making sure your child is able to open it and close it at home is crucial to lunchtime success. If you need help choosing a container that is right for your child, head over to MOMables.com to see the ones I recommend.

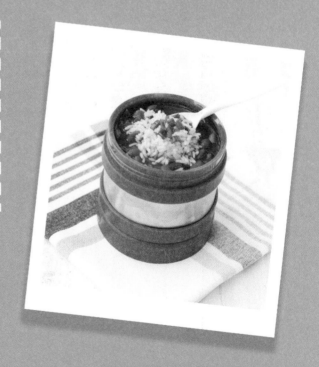

CRAFTING A HEALTHY LUNCHBOX

The recipes in this book are not designed to contain an exact ratio of protein to carbohydrates to fats. They were not calculated in some lab to exact proportion to the "average" child. Instead, they were created in my kitchen and tested by thousands of kids in my community. Because, as you and I know, no two kids are alike.

That said, the recipes you'll find in these pages *are* health-focused and consciously crafted. For those of you who need me to be a "little more specific," you'll find that these lunchboxes contain the following elements:

- Protein-rich foods
- Carbohydrates or starches
- An assortment of color
- Fruit and vegetables
- Water

Let's quickly cover each of these categories and how/why I find them important. Rest assured, the bottom line here is filling up your child (and mine!) with the best balance of health and taste as possible!

Protein-Rich Foods

Foods high in protein are vital for our kid's growth and brain development. Protein doesn't always have to come from an animal source. In fact, in this book, I have many vegetarian protein-rich lunches, such as the Honey Bee Sandwich (page 51), Hummus Avocado Sandwich (page 52), Hummus Monster (page 75), Lunchbox Falafels (page 115), and the Southwest Quinoa (page 157).

Carbohydrates

Carbohydrates provide our kids with a steady stream of energy to help their sugar levels stay balanced. Whole-grain carbohydrates are best, so I suggest you fill your pantry with an assortment of them. Whole grains also contain fiber, something kids (and adults) often don't get enough of in their diets.

Note that the more processed the food, the less original whole grains, fiber, and nutrients it will contain (many of these are added in during processing but tend to lack real nutrition).

An Assortment of Color

Kids love rainbows. I am a firm believer that a lunch that is built on a variety of foods will have lots of color and kid appeal. When kids *eat* their homemade lunch, that's success in my book.

Fruits and Vegetables

We've all heard the daily recommendation to eat five servings of fruits and vegetables, but perhaps not everyone realizes how many different ways there are to get them in!

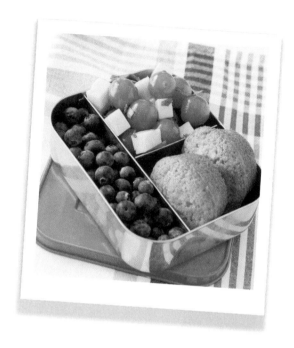

Fruits and vegetables are a great fresh source of vitamins, minerals, and fiber. While it's okay to supplement our kids' diets with a multivitamin, you're much better off incorporating more of those nutrients through fresh foods.

If your child is a picky eater and will only eat one or two types of fruits or vegetables, don't give yourself a hard time. Serve those fresh and incorporate new ones through the recipes from this book! Smoothies, for example, are the perfect vessel to add more fruit, and quiches, frittatas, and tomato sauce are all ideal places to sneak in more veggies. Don't worry; I've got you fully covered in this book.

Water

Every day, I send my kids with a stainless steel thermos filled with fresh, cool water. On occasion, I add a spoonful or two of 100 percent pomegranate juice or apple cider for added flavor. In winter, I like to add my vitamin C cubes (page 190) for a little added immunity boost.

A Few Other Items

This isn't a low-salt, low-fat, low-carb, low-everything cookbook—this is a fresh-food-made-of-real-ingredients type of cookbook. That said, I am mindful of keeping everything in moderation (salt, sugar, and fat included) and will expand a bit more on that here.

Salt

Sadly, many kids are eating far more salt in their diet than recommended. This is primarily because of processed foods, where high levels of sodium often hide. Foods labeled "reduced sodium" contain at least 25 percent less *than the original version*, so while they may be a bit healthier, they're not necessarily so.

When you can, opt for fresh or frozen vegetables instead of canned, which may contain added salt. If you use canned beans, be sure to rinse them before consuming them. With the exception of baking, you can usually reduce the amount of salt called for in recipes (if you're strict about a low-sodium diet) and still yield good results.

Sugars

Like salt, sugar is added to processed foods in many different forms. It's also often found in low-fat or reduced-fat versions of many foods, where the sugar content has often been increased to make up for the fat/flavor taken out (a slippery slope to be sure).

It's easy to say no to sodas, but oftentimes we forget that a few glasses of juice, a slice of cake, and sugary yogurts can add up too. The good news is that when you begin to rely on fresh foods to build your child's lunch and keep treats to a minimum, you help control sugar intake and keep it in moderation.

Try to make your own Rainbow Fruit Cups (page 202) instead of buying those with fruit soaked in sugary syrup. When you can, opt for making your own baked goods and treats, because these often have less sugar per serving than the packaged version.

Fats

Kids need some fats in their diet for optimal health, which is why I suggest adding good fats into your diet whenever possible. Most of these good fats come from good-for-you foods such as avocados, nuts, and seeds, and certain oils, such as coconut oil and olive oil.

Whenever possible, I opt for the real thing when cooking and baking, because many of the alternatives have a long list of unidentifiable ingredients or are processed foods in disguise.

Introducing Real Foods to Your Family

Feeding my family real foods was a challenge at first. My kids were resistant, and I was used to being a short-order cook. Remember, your job is to provide your children with nutritious foods; it's their choice to eat them or not. Below are some of the things that have worked for me.

INTRODUCE ONE NEW HEALTHY FOOD A WEEK

If your kids (and husband) aren't used to healthier versions of old favorites, start slowly. Pick one recipe in this book, modify it for allergies or preferences, and take it from there. Showing your family that you are committed to providing healthier choices is very important. Plus, one new thing per week keeps it simple for you!

TAKE YOUR KIDS GROCERY SHOPPING

As a mom, I dread dragging my three children to the grocery store each week, so I take turns bringing one with me, and I ask them to pick out a healthy fruit or veggie they might want to try this week. When they say they don't want anything new, I suggest that if they choose it, it's a lot better than mom's mystery ingredient.

GO 50/50 WITH WHOLE GRAINS

When I tried to serve my kids whole wheat pasta, they complained that it was chewy and rubbery. I decided to mix half whole wheat with half white pasta at first, before transitioning to 100 percent whole wheat, which they are now fine with. Some brands of pasta even contain a 50/50 mix, so the work's already done for you!

MAKE A STORE-BOUGHT FAVORITE HOMEMADE

Two of my go-to lunchbox recipes are the Homemade O's (page 145) and Homemade Ramen (page 151). These two recipes are incredibly easy to make and so much healthier! You'll also find things such as homemade breads, Lunchbox Granola (page 44), Lunchbox Cheese Crackers (page 192), Chocolate Athlete Bars (page 195), and so many more! Many of these recipes are the perfect gateway to getting your kids involved in the kitchen.

ADD THE NEW WITH THE OLD

Adding new foods is simpler than you might think. Master a kid-friendly recipe, such as Mini Quiches (page 125), and add other veggies to it. Another fun way to introduce new fruits is with the Rainbow Fruit Cups (page 202). Make this recipe with two or three of your child's favorite fruits, and add one new one. Soon you'll have a list of new foods your kids will eat!

Mastering the Kitchen: Cook Once, Eat Twice, and Other Tips

Whipping up dinner in less than thirty minutes can be tough when you have kids to bathe or are still waiting for soccer practice to end. And don't get me started on how tough it is to make lunches in the morning when the coffee pot hasn't had time to finish brewing. This is nearly impossible for me to do! I'm just not a morning person, seriously.

A few years ago, faced with daily kitchen chores while holding a six-month-old baby in my arms and a twenty-month-old toddler clinging to my leg, I decided to streamline my kitchen routines. I told myself this: Whatever I cook tonight must yield enough for another meal and lunch! *Cook once, eat (at least) twice.* Boil extra pasta, cook extra rice, roast an extra chicken, double the recipe for the Veggie Tomato Sauce (on page 144) and freeze it for a later meal. *Voila!*

Aside from my big-batch advice, here are a few additional tips for feeding your family real food while still managing a busy life.

MAKE A PLAN

Spend twenty minutes a week writing down the recipes and ingredients you'll need for the week. Having everything on hand allows you to execute your plan throughout the week. If you need help, subscribing to a meal planning website will help you get started.

HAVE HEALTHY SNACKS READY TO GO

Many of the snack recipes in this book can be made in larger batches and individually packaged. Place a basket in your pantry labeled "snacks" with individual servings of portable goodies. Check out the "Healthy Snacks on the Go" section (page 221) for tips on how to package them individually.

MAKE THE FREEZER YOUR FRIEND

Making sure your kids eat breakfast can be difficult when you are rushing out the door. Designate one evening per month to double or triple (or more!) some of the breakfast recipes in this book. Cook or bake them, freeze, and have them ready to go for busy mornings.

PREP EARLY

Wash your produce, marinade meat inside a large ziplock bag, and begin prepping some recipes. Any chopping, mixing, or marinating you can do ahead of time will surely save you time later. You can also prep tomorrow's breakfast and lunches prior to cleaning up the kitchen from dinner. It's already a mess!

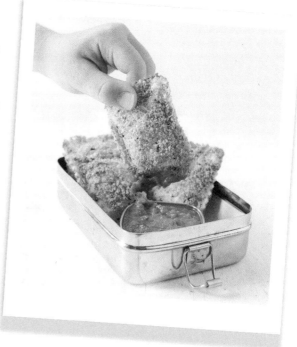

On to the Recipes!

The recipes in this book were designed with busy parents in mind. As a full-time working mom of three kids, I don't want to stare at the refrigerator every morning, waiting for the food to call out and say, "Take me! I'm what you've been looking for to build a lunchbox today!"

Nearly all the recipes in this book can be made ahead of time, or at least, preassembled so that all you have to do is warm them up in the morning. You'll see my little "Laura's Tips" throughout the book as well, which share insights gained after testing thousands of recipes and packing nearly as many lunchboxes.

Remember that the ingredients in most recipes are not set in stone. If your child prefers mozzarella instead of Cheddar cheese, go ahead and swap it out. The baking recipes, however, will yield the most delicious results when you follow the recipe as is and minimize substitutions. Either way, this is a great start for your family.

DIETARY RESTRICTIONS AND SUBSTITUTIONS

The best recipes are those that are flexible enough to accommodate ingredient swaps and adjust for food allergies and intolerances.

Many of the recipes in this book are naturally gluten-free, nut-free, soy-free, corn-free, and dairy-free. Some, however, you'll have to use as a foundation and make it your own. Nearly all the recipes in this book can be adapted, with the exception of the baked goods.

You can purchase gluten-free breads, pastas, and many other products at regular grocery stores. Use those when a recipe calls for whole grain or whole wheat breads and pastas.

Making dairy-free adjustments can be a bit trickier, since oftentimes cheese is used to bind and hold together the ingredients, a grilled sandwich, for example. However, many of the recipes are delicious on their own, where cheese is just an add-on. For my youngest child, who is mostly dairy-free, I use a nondairy cream cheese spread alternative on occasion. Or, I make my own version with nuts.

Finally, if you have a child with nut allergies, or your kids attend a school that is nut-free, you can purchase nut-free butters at nearly all grocery stores. Nut-free butters are made of sunflower seeds, soy, or yellow peas.

Let's Get Started!

If you want to learn to make school lunch favorites from scratch, this book gives you a lot of opportunities. If you want to just try a few things and slowly work up to all homemade, you can easily do that too! This is a no-judgment zone!

Don't know where to begin? Pick an item, or food group, that your child consumes a lot of (hint: go look in your pantry), and learn how to make one thing within that category homemade (crackers, for instance). After that, purchase items to go with those with the shortest ingredient list possible (fresh cheese, for instance). It's that easy!

Packing the best school lunches for your child shouldn't require you to slave in the kitchen. Making a new thing from scratch, trying new recipes, and getting your kids involved—that's all part of building a better lunchbox!

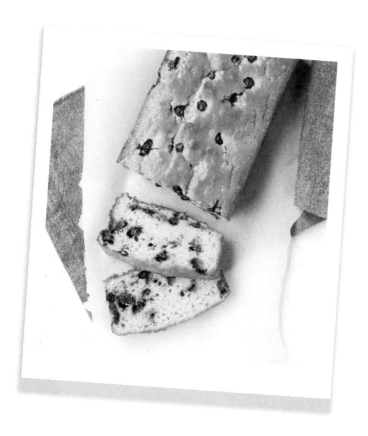

CHAPTER 2

GET OUT THE DOOR: BREAKFASTS TO GO

My kids are *turtle* slow in the morning, so by the time they sit down for breakfast it's nearly always time to go!

Growing tired of half-eaten bagels and soggy pancakes, one day, I decided to fill an empty lunch container with their breakfast. If the kids were able to finish their breakfast at the table, great. If not, they could easily take it to-go!

The recipes included in this section are portable, delicious, and kid-approved. They are also the building blocks of some of our fun breakfast lunches.

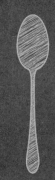

Perfect Pancakes

I have my Auntie Colleen to thank for this recipe. Once, while staying at her house, she made these beautiful pancakes with fresh blueberries from her farmers' market. They were fluffy, not overly sweet, and easy to make—simply amazing! Of course, I asked her for the recipe, and 15 years later, I am still making these at least once a week.

1½ cups (200 g) all-purpose flour

3½ teaspoons (16 g) baking powder

1 teaspoon salt

1 tablespoon (13 g) sugar

1¼ cups (294 ml) milk

1 egg

3 tablespoons (42 g) butter, melted (optional), plus more for serving

Maple syrup, for serving

In a large bowl, sift together the flour, baking powder, salt, and sugar. Make a well (or volcano, as my son calls it) in the middle, and pour in the milk, egg, and melted butter, if using; mix with a fork or whisk until smooth.

Heat a griddle or large pan over medium-high heat (I set my griddle at 375°F [190°C]).

Pour or scoop ¼ cup (125 g) of batter for each pancake. Wait until bubbles form on the top to flip. Brown on the other side and serve with butter and maple syrup.

YIELD: 10 pancakes

Kitchen Notes

To substitute or make with:

- **100 percent whole wheat flour:** Add an additional teaspoon of baking powder and an additional tablespoon (15 ml) of milk.

- **50 percent whole wheat flour (half all-purpose, half whole wheat):** Add ½ teaspoon baking powder.

- **Gluten-Free Flour Mix:** Use a 1:1 substitution ratio for the flour. For optimal results, I suggest King Arthur Flour Gluten Free All-Purpose Mix

- **Flax:** Add ¼ cup (28 g) ground flax and remove ¼ cup (31 g) flour; add ½ teaspoon baking powder.

You can also add 1 medium mashed banana or up to 1 cup (155 g) blueberries or nuts to the original recipe or one of the variations above.

I also love to double or triple this recipe and substitute the pancakes for bread in school lunches. Store the extra batches in the freezer so you can grab them whenever needed.

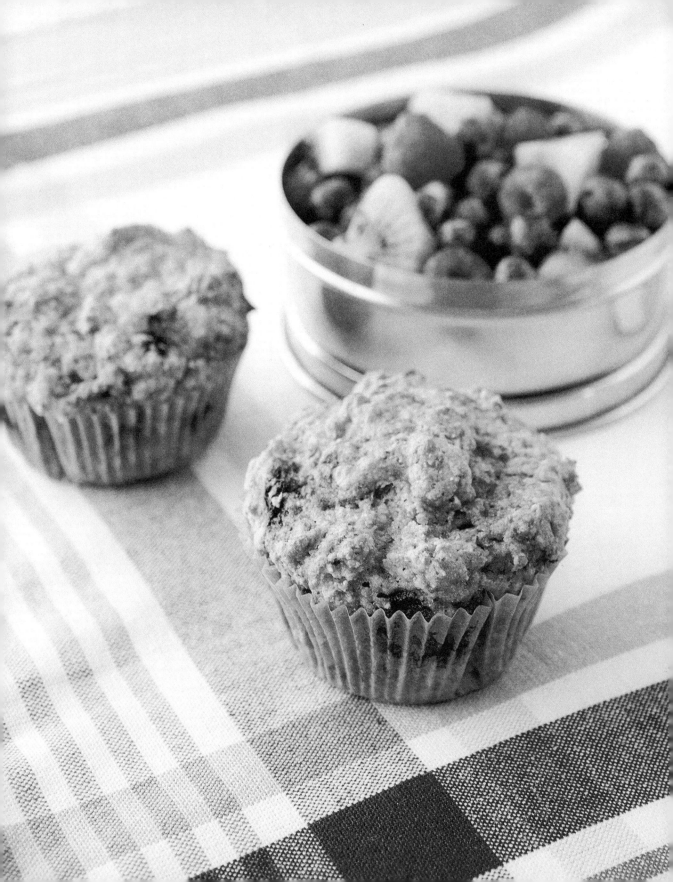

kitchen Sink Muffins

My favorite kinds of recipes are those that are flexible and will yield delicious results. Recipes that, on any given day, I can make work with what I might have in my pantry. These muffins are just that kind of recipe. When you mix and match any of the add-ins, even your pickiest eater is sure to find a combination that they will love.

For Muffins:

2 cups (250 g) whole wheat pastry flour

2 tablespoons (14 g) ground flax meal

2 teaspoons (9 g) baking powder

1 teaspoon baking soda

⅓ cup (67 g) granulated sugar

1 cup (245 g) unsweetened applesauce

2 tablespoons (28 g) melted butter

⅓ cup (78 ml) milk

For Add-Ins:

1 cup (155 g) fresh or frozen fruit, such as blueberries, thawed

½ cup (55 g) pecans, walnuts, or almonds, chopped

⅔ cup (97 g) dried fruit, such as raisins

1 teaspoon (3 g) ground cinnamon

1 cup (175 g) semi-sweet chocolate chips

Preheat the oven to 400°F (200°C) and line a standard-size muffin pan with liners.

In a large mixing bowl, combine the dry ingredients. Add in the applesauce, melted butter, and milk, and stir until thoroughly combined, creating a smooth, stiff batter.

Gently fold in the add-ins, if using, and then divide the batter equally, spooning it into the muffin cups.

Bake the muffins for 15 to 20 minutes, or until the tops are golden. Transfer to a cooling rack. Serve warm or at room temperature. Store the remaining muffins in an airtight container.

YIELD: 12 muffins

Laura's Tip

You can freeze muffins after they are baked and cooled for future grab-and-go breakfasts. To rewarm, heat the muffin for 10 to 15 seconds in the microwave.

Eggs-to-Go

There is no such thing as "no time for breakfast" when you have a pan of these ready to go in your fridge!

12 eggs

¾ cup (175 ml) milk

Veggies (green and red bell peppers, onions, mushrooms, tomatoes, etc.), chopped

Meat (diced ham, turkey sausage, bacon, etc.)

Shredded Cheddar cheese (for topping)

Preheat the oven to 375°F (190°C) and grease or spray a standard 12-cup muffin tin.

In a large bowl, whisk the eggs and milk. Pour the egg mixture evenly into the greased wells until each well is about half full. Add in the veggies, and top with the meat and cheese.

Top off each well with the additional egg mixture (being careful to leave a little room at the top), and bake for 18 to 20 minutes.

Remove from the oven, pop them out of each well, and serve. Allow extras to cool before storing in the refrigerator.

YIELD: 12 servings

Breakfast Burrito ▶

No more frozen breakfast burritos with mystery ingredients, or a quick trip to the drive-through. This is the perfect make-ahead recipe that your entire family will love!

1 tablespoon (16 g) Homemade Salsa (page 180)

1 tablespoon (15 g) sour cream

One 8-inch (20 cm) tortilla

1 large egg, scrambled

2 tablespoons (15 g) shredded cheese

1 slice (7 g) bacon, cooked and crumbled

In a small bowl, the mix salsa and sour cream.

Lay the tortilla on a cutting board, and spread the salsa mixture evenly on the middle third. Lay the egg, cheese, and bacon on top. Fold the sides in, and then roll into a burrito.

For the lunchbox: Wrap in parchment paper and a thin layer of foil to retain the heat (optional). If you must have these warm, cut them in half and insert face up inside a thermos.

YIELD: 1 serving

Kitchen Note

Get a pack (or two) of flour tortillas and make extra breakfast burritos. Line a baking sheet with parchment paper, lay the burritos flat 1 inch (2.5 cm) apart and flash freeze. Transfer the frozen burritos into a freezer ziplock bag. To warm, microwave for 30 seconds to 1 minute and enjoy. Store in the freezer up to 2 months.

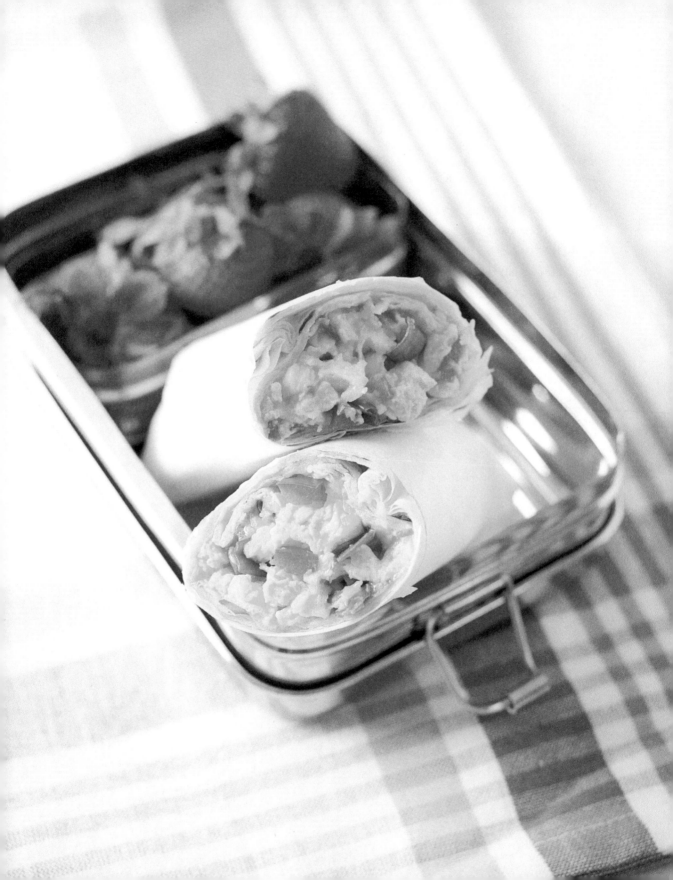

Breakfast Cookies

"If it looks like a cookie and tastes like a cookie, then it must be a cookie!" said Cookie Monster on *Sesame Street*. It is—sort of. Little do my kids know that these "cookies" have protein, fiber, vitamins, minerals, and omega 3s.

1 large banana, mashed

½ cup (130 g) peanut butter

½ cup (170 g) honey

2 teaspoons (10 ml) vanilla extract

1 cup (80 g) old-fashioned oats

¼ cup (31 g) whole wheat flour

¼ cup (28 g) ground flaxseed

¼ cup (32 g) powdered milk or vanilla protein

2 teaspoons (5 g) ground cinnamon

½ teaspoon baking soda

¾ cup (110 g) add-ins: raisins, chocolate chips, and/or dried fruit

Preheat the oven to 350°F (180°C) and line two cookie sheets with parchment paper.

In the bowl of your stand mixer, or a large bowl, mix the banana, peanut butter, honey, and vanilla.

In a small bowl, combine the oats, flour, flax, powdered milk, cinnamon, and baking soda.

Slowly add the dry mixture to the wet ingredients, mixing until everything is combined evenly. Fold in your add-ins, up to ¾ cup (110 g).

Using a ¼ cup (60 g) measuring cup or scoop, drop dough scoops 3 inches (7.5 cm) apart onto your lined baking sheets. Using your hands, flatten your dough scoops to about ½-inch (1.25 cm) tall. This will ensure even baking.

Bake the cookies for 15 minutes, or until lightly browned. Allow the cookies to cool for 5 minutes on the baking sheet before transferring to a wire rack to cool completely.

Store in an airtight container or resealable plastic bag for up to 3 days or freeze for up to 2 months; thaw before serving.

YIELD: 12 cookies

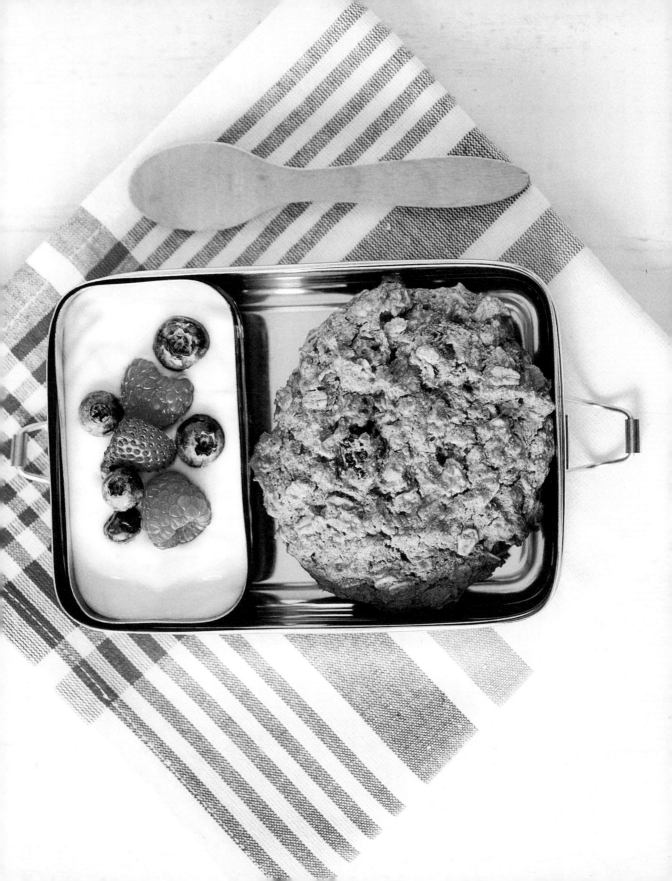

French Toast Stix

Breakfast for dinner is my kids' favorite, so why not serve breakfast for lunch? You'll rock their lunchbox with these delicious sticks of cinnamon goodness! You can make extras and store in the freezer for a quick breakfast too.

2 eggs

¼ cup (60 ml) milk

½ teaspoon vanilla extract

4 slices cinnamon raisin bread

Butter or butter spray for cooking

2 tablespoons (30 ml) maple syrup, for dipping

In a shallow bowl or baking dish, whisk together the eggs, milk, and vanilla. Add the bread slices and let soak, turning once or twice, until all of the egg mixture has been absorbed (about 3 minutes).

Heat a large nonstick skillet or griddle over medium heat, and spread or spray the butter evenly over the pan bottom.

Add the soaked bread slices side by side. Cook until the bottoms are golden, about 2 minutes. Carefully flip them over. Cook until the second side is also golden and the centers puff slightly, about 2 more minutes.

Cut into strips for dipping, and serve with a side of maple syrup stored in a small container with a lid.

YIELD: 2 servings

Kitchen Note

Make these the night before, and warm them in the morning before packing for school.

Cinnamon Roll Overnight Oatmeal

My husband calls oatmeal a "stick to your belly" breakfast. It's filling, hearty, and budget-friendly. This version cooks itself while your family sleeps, and in the morning, the house smells amazing!

1 cup (80 g) old-fashioned oats

4 cups (950 ml) water

½ cup (120 ml) milk

¼ cup (60 g) packed brown sugar

½ teaspoon vanilla extract

1 teaspoon cinnamon

Maple syrup, for serving

Milk, for serving

Add all ingredients (except maple syrup and milk) into a small crockpot. Cook on low for 6 hours.

Serve with the maple syrup and milk.

YIELD: 3 servings

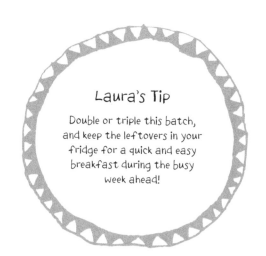

Laura's Tip

Double or triple this batch, and keep the leftovers in your fridge for a quick and easy breakfast during the busy week ahead!

Chocolate Chip Freezer Scones

I became addicted to these scones after trying a recipe from the Culinary Institute of America. I use their basic recipe as a guide, adjusting it to suit my kids' taste preferences—adding chocolate, of course!

3 cups (375 g) all-purpose flour

½ cup (100 g) plus 3 tablespoons (40 g) sugar, divided

2 tablespoons (28 g) baking powder

½ teaspoon salt

½ cup (88 g) chocolate chips

2 cups (475 ml) heavy cream or half and half

2 tablespoons (30 ml) milk

Line a baking sheet with parchment paper.

Sift the flour into a mixing bowl, then add ½ cup (100 g) sugar, baking powder, salt, and chocolate chips.

Make a well in the center of the flour mixture (or a volcano, as my son likes to call it). Add the cream to the well, and mix with a wooden spoon, or using your hands, until the batter is evenly moistened. The dough will be a bit sticky.

Using your hands, make twelve 2-inch (5 cm) scones and place them onto the baking sheet. If the dough sticks to your hands, rub a little flour on them. Place the baking sheet in the freezer for about 2 hours, until the dough is frozen, or overnight to prevent them from "melting" when they are baked.

Preheat the oven to 350°F (180°C). Remove the baking sheet from the freezer and let the scones thaw for about 5 minutes. If you are baking all 12 scones, you will need to line a second cookie sheet and separate, because they will expand while baking. Otherwise, place the ones you don't need inside a freezer bag, and put them back in the freezer for another day.

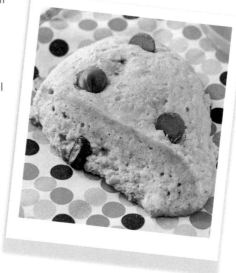

Brush the scones with the milk and sprinkle with the additional 3 tablespoons (40 g) of reserved sugar.

Bake the scones until golden brown, about 30 to 40 minutes. Allow to cool on the baking sheet for a few minutes, then transfer to a wire rack to continue cooling.

Enjoy the same day they are made, or freeze for up to 4 weeks.

YIELD: 12 scones

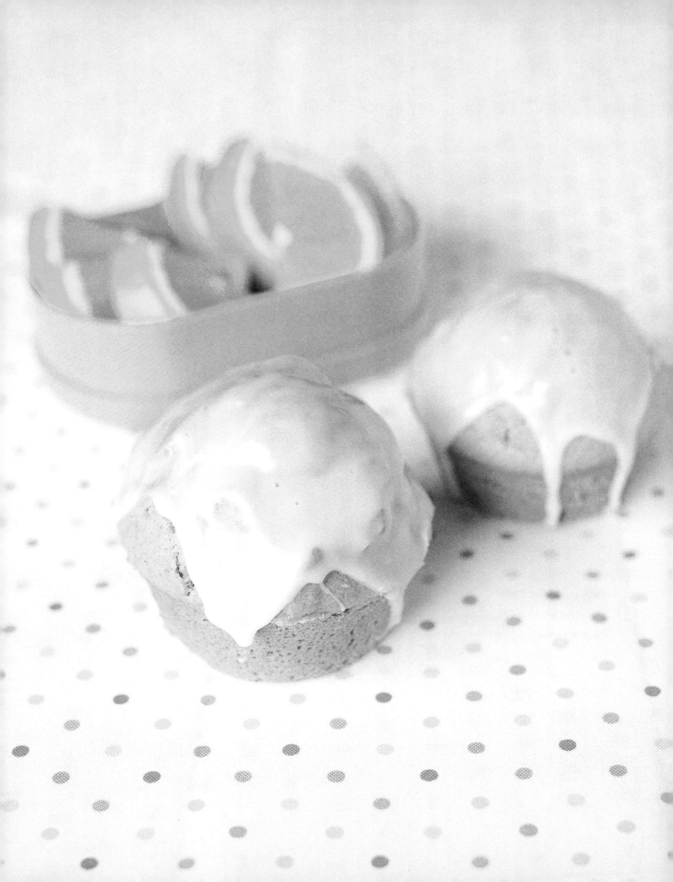

Glazed Cake Donut Muffins

What do you get when you want to satisfy your kid's donut craving, don't own a donut pan, and want a healthier version? These Glazed Cake Donut Muffins of course! Don't let the word "donut" fool you; these are okay to have for breakfast—on occasion.

For Muffins:

¼ cup (56 g) butter, softened

½ cup (100 g) evaporated cane sugar

⅓ cup (50 g) brown sugar

2 large eggs

¼ cup (61 g) applesauce

2 teaspoons (10 ml) vanilla extract

1½ teaspoons baking powder

¼ teaspoon baking soda

1 teaspoon ground cinnamon

¾ teaspoon salt

2⅔ cups (320 g) whole wheat pastry flour (or all-purpose flour)

1 cup (235 ml) milk

For Glaze:

¼ cup (60 ml) milk

1 teaspoon vanilla extract

2 cups (240 g) confectioners' sugar

Preheat the oven to 400°F (200°C) and lightly grease a large or standard muffin pan, or line with cups.

To make the muffins: In the bowl of your stand mixer, or a medium-size bowl, cream together the butter and sugars until smooth. Add the eggs, applesauce, and vanilla, mixing to combine. Add the baking powder, baking soda, cinnamon, and salt, mixing on low to combine.

Slowly add the flour into the mixture in three additions, adding alternately with the milk (beginning and ending with the flour), until everything is thoroughly combined.

Spoon the thick batter evenly into the prepared pan, filling the cups nearly full.

Bake the muffins for 17 to 20 minutes, or until the muffins are a pale golden brown and a toothpick inserted in the center comes out clean. Cool on a wire rack.

To make the glaze: In a medium bowl, combine all the ingredients and stir until smooth.

Dip the top of the muffins into the glaze after they have cooled for several minutes. Serve warm, or cool on a rack and place in an airtight container. Store for a day or so at room temperature.

YIELD: 12 large muffins or 18 cupcake-size muffins

Lunchbox Granola

Once you learn how to make your own granola, you'll never buy store-bought again. It's great for breakfast, as a snack, or in the lunchbox.

6 cups (480 g) old-fashioned oats

1½ cups (218 g) nuts (slivered almonds, pumpkin seeds, walnuts, etc.)

1 cup (80 g) shredded sweet coconut

½ cup (73 g) whole flaxseeds

1½ cups (218 g) raisins, cranberries, or dried fruit

½ cup (120 ml) plus 2 tablespoons (30 ml) maple syrup

½ cup (75 g) brown sugar

½ cup (120 ml) coconut oil (melted), butter (melted), or vegetable oil

¾ teaspoon salt

Preheat the oven to 250°F (120°C).

In a large bowl, combine the dry ingredients.

In a separate bowl, combine the maple syrup, brown sugar, oil, and salt.

Add the wet ingredients to the dry and mix well (using your hands if needed), until all is evenly coated.

Divide the granola mixture onto 2 sheet pans. Cook for 50 minutes, stirring every 15 to 20 minutes, to achieve an even color.

YIELD: About 8 cups

Whole Wheat Waffles

Dust off your waffle maker because your kids are going to love this wholesome breakfast staple.

½ cup (120 ml) warm water

3 tablespoons (21 g) ground flaxseed

6 tablespoons (90 g) butter, melted

1½ cups (355 ml) milk

1¾ cups (210 g) whole wheat pastry flour (all-purpose flour may be substituted)

1 tablespoon (14 g) baking powder

1 tablespoon (13 g) granulated sugar (optional)

Pinch of salt

Preheat your waffle maker.

In a medium bowl, mix the water and flaxseed. Let it rest for a few minutes, or until it has become thick in consistency. Add the butter and milk, and mix to combine.

In a large bowl, combine the dry ingredients. Make a well in the center, and pour in the milk mixture. Stir until just combined, because over-stirred batter can make for tough, rubbery waffles. A few lumps are okay.

Spoon a scoopful of batter onto each waffle grid. Spread the batter to within ¼ inch of the edge of the grids. Close the lid and bake until the waffle is golden brown.

YIELD: 4 to 6 waffles—sizes vary by waffle maker

CHAPTER 3

FILL THE BOX: SANDWICHES AND MORE

I like to think of sandwiches as the main course of any lunchbox. Yet, long gone are the days when I packed a plain ham and cheese, or a peanut butter and jelly, more than once a week.

The sandwiches, wraps, and pinwheels in this book incorporate dinner leftovers, easy-to-find ingredients, and kid-friendly combinations.

I promise: After you try these recipes, your kids will never think of a sandwich as a boring lunch option ever again.

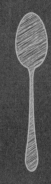

Avocado Bacon Melt

When my son wouldn't try avocado, I was crushed. He said he didn't like the "cold and slimy green thing." Short of bribing him with a sweet treat, I decided to grill it, add bacon and cheese, and give it another try. He loved it. Kids—they are funny like that.

¼ avocado, mashed

2 slices (15 g) bacon, cooked and finely chopped

2 slices whole-grain bread

Olive oil, for grilling

2 slices (40 g) provolone cheese

In a small bowl, combine the avocado and bacon.

Lay the bread slices on a cutting board. Butter or brush the outside of the bread slices with the oil. Flip them over.

Top one bread slice with provolone cheese, then place the bacon-avocado mixture on top. Top with the remaining cheese and bread slice.

Grill the sandwich on a preheated panini grill, or in a skillet over medium heat, for 3 to 4 minutes until golden brown and the cheese is melted (if using a skillet, flip halfway through).

YIELD: 1 serving

Grilled Taco Sandwich

I always seem to have leftover taco meat from Taco Tuesdays at my house. I couldn't think of a better way to repurpose it than this, and it has become a kid favorite.

Butter, for grilling

2 slices whole-grain bread

2 slices (40 g) Cheddar cheese

2 tablespoons (25 g) cooked ground beef

1 tablespoon (6 g) black olives, sliced

¼ cup (65 g) Homemade Salsa, for dipping (page 180)

Butter one side of both bread slices, then flip over onto a cutting board. Place cheese on top of both bread slices, top one slice with ground beef and olives, and close the sandwich.

Place the sandwich in a skillet over medium heat. Grill for 2 to 3 minutes, until the cheese has begun to melt and the bread is golden brown. Press down with a spatula, flip, and grill the second side. Remove from the pan onto a cutting board.

Allow the grilled sandwich to cool down for 5 minutes before packing in a lunch container.

Serve with ¼ cup (65 g) Homemade Salsa (page 180) for dipping.

YIELD: 1 serving

Pretzelwich

My daughter says that everything tastes better in a pretzel roll. Her happy empty lunchbox proves it's true.

1 teaspoon mustard

2 teaspoons (9 g) mayonnaise

1 pretzel roll, sliced in half

2 slices (40 g) ham

1 slice (20 g) provolone cheese

Lettuce (optional)

Tomato (optional)

Mix mustard and mayonnaise, and spread onto both sides of the roll. Layer the ham and cheese, top with the lettuce and tomato, if using, and close the pretzelwich.

YIELD: 1 serving

Egg Salad Sandwich

I usually hard-boil about a half-dozen eggs at the beginning of the week and keep them in my fridge, just in case we need to assemble an extra lunch quickly, or add protein to a veggie-laden meal.

1 hard-boiled egg, mashed or chopped

2 teaspoons (10 g) plain Greek yogurt or mayonnaise

Dash of ground paprika

Salt and pepper

2 slices whole-grain bread

In a small bowl, combine the egg, yogurt, and paprika until well combined. Season with the salt and pepper to taste.

Spread the egg salad on one of the bread slices, and close the sandwich.

YIELD: 1 sandwich

Kitchen Note

I make this sandwich the night before. In the morning, I place it inside the freezer for 20 minutes while I get the kids ready. This extra cooling helps the egg salad stay cold inside the lunchbox, and I don't need to bother with extra ice packs.

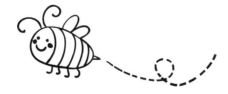

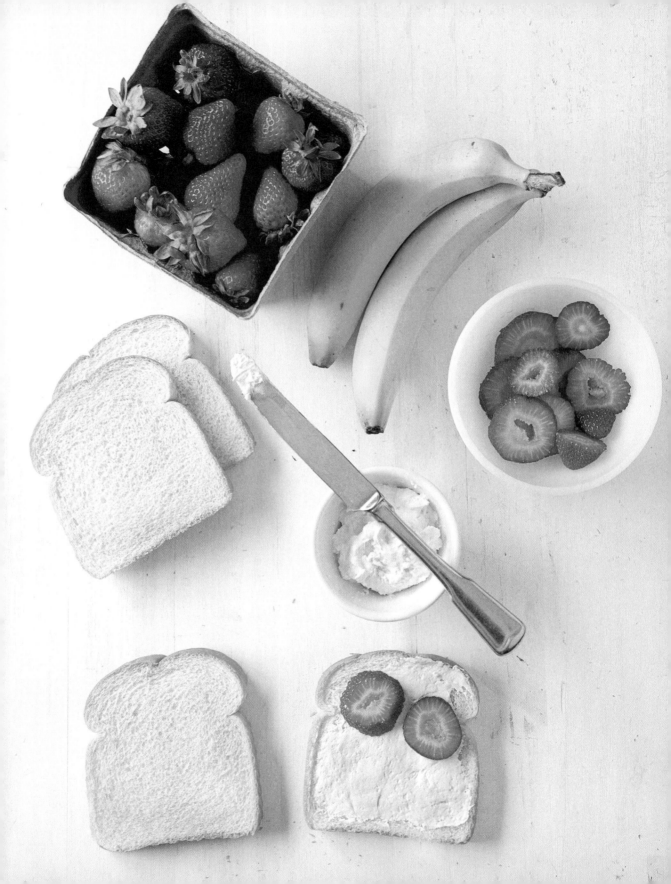

◄ Angel Food Sandwich

The first time I made this sandwich, my daughter said: "Mom, I am quite sure this is what angels eat in heaven."

1½ tablespoons (23 g) whipped cream cheese

2 slices white wheat sandwich bread

½ small banana, sliced

1 or 2 strawberries, sliced

Spread the cream cheese evenly on each slice of bread.

Layer with the banana and strawberries, and close the sandwich.

YIELD: 1 serving

Candy Apple Sandwich

Healthier and more nutritious than the red-sugar coated ones and way less sticky!

2 tablespoons (32 g) Caramel Peanut Butter (page 171)

2 slices whole-grain bread

¼ apple, sliced thin

Spread the peanut butter on both slices of bread. Lay the apple slices evenly over one of the slices, and close the sandwich.

YIELD: 1 serving

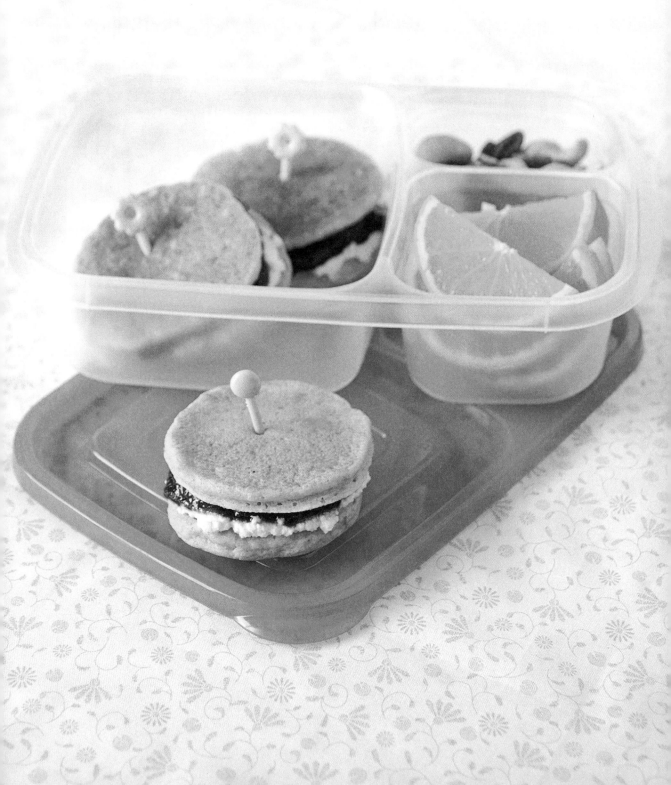

◄ Ricotta and Jam Pancake Sandwich

Your kids will love opening up their lunchboxes and seeing that their sandwiches are made with pancakes.

3 tablespoons (28 g) part-skim ricotta cheese

4 Perfect Pancakes (page 33), 2-inch (5 cm) diameter

1 tablespoon (20 g) Easy Freezer Jam (page 170)

Spread the ricotta evenly onto two of the pancakes; top with the jam, then top with the remaining pancakes.

YIELD: 1 serving

Honey Bee Sandwich

"Creamy, sweet, and delicious" is how my son describes this sandwich. Loaded with protein and whole grains, it makes this mom happy.

3 tablespoons (49 g) part-skim ricotta cheese

2 slices hearty oat bread, lightly toasted

1 teaspoon honey

Spread the ricotta on one slice of bread and drizzle with the honey. Top with the other slice of bread.

YIELD: 1 serving

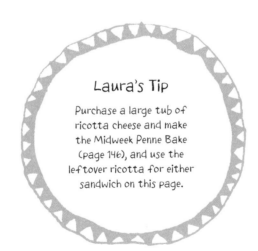

Laura's Tip

Purchase a large tub of ricotta cheese and make the Midweek Penne Bake (page 146), and use the leftover ricotta for either sandwich on this page.

Hummus Avocado Sandwich

I call this the "power sandwich." Easy to assemble and loaded with nutrition, it's the perfect sandwich for active kids.

2 slices multi-grain bread

2 tablespoons (30 g) hummus

¼ avocado, sliced

Lay the bread on a cutting board and spread the hummus over each slice.

Top one slice with the avocado, and close the sandwich.

YIELD: 1 serving

Grilled Harvest Sandwich

My friend Alison introduced me to this grilled Cheddar and apple sandwich. While I'm a huge fan of juicy and sweet apples on their own, I think this grilled cheese sandwich might be my favorite savory way to enjoy them!

Butter or oil, for grilling

2 slices bread

½ teaspoon spicy mustard (optional)

1 apple, any variety, thinly sliced

1 or 2 slices Cheddar cheese

Preheat the skillet or griddle over medium heat. Butter one side of a slice of the bread. Place the bread, buttered side down, into the skillet and spread the spicy mustard, if using, on the top. Distribute the apple slices and cheese, using enough to cover the entire surface area of the bread.

Butter the second slice of bread on one side, and place, buttered side up, on top of the sandwich.

Grill until lightly browned and flip over. Continue grilling until the cheese is melted and the second side is golden brown. Slice in half and serve immediately.

For a school lunch: Allow the sandwich to cool on a cooling rack or cutting board before placing it inside a lunch container (this prevents the bread from getting mushy).

YIELD: 1 serving

The Frenchman

The only thing better than finding this sandwich in the lunchbox is eating it at a café in Paris. But this brings a little taste of France home all the same!

One 3- to 4-inch (7.5 to 10 cm) piece French baguette

2 teaspoons (9 g) mayonnaise

3 slices (60 g) ham

1½ ounces (30 g) Brie, sliced thin

Using a serrated knife, slice the baguette across the middle.

Spread the mayonnaise, top with the ham and Brie, and close the sandwich.

YIELD: 1 sandwich

Kitchen Note

If you have a panini press, this sandwich will magically melt together and truly bring out the Brie flavors. It also makes the crust crispy and delicious.

Boy Meets Girl Sandwich

My five-year-old son once told me that strawberries are for girls. His sister, who doesn't eat peanut butter, happens to love strawberries. Oddly enough, I put the two ingredients together only to find they both love this combination!

2 tablespoons (32 g) peanut butter

2 slices whole-grain sandwich bread

¼ cup (40 g) strawberries, sliced

Dash of cinnamon (optional)

Spread peanut butter on both bread slices, layer the strawberries, sprinkle with the cinnamon, if using, and close the sandwich.

YIELD: 1 serving

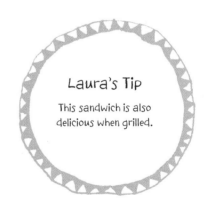

Laura's Tip

This sandwich is also delicious when grilled.

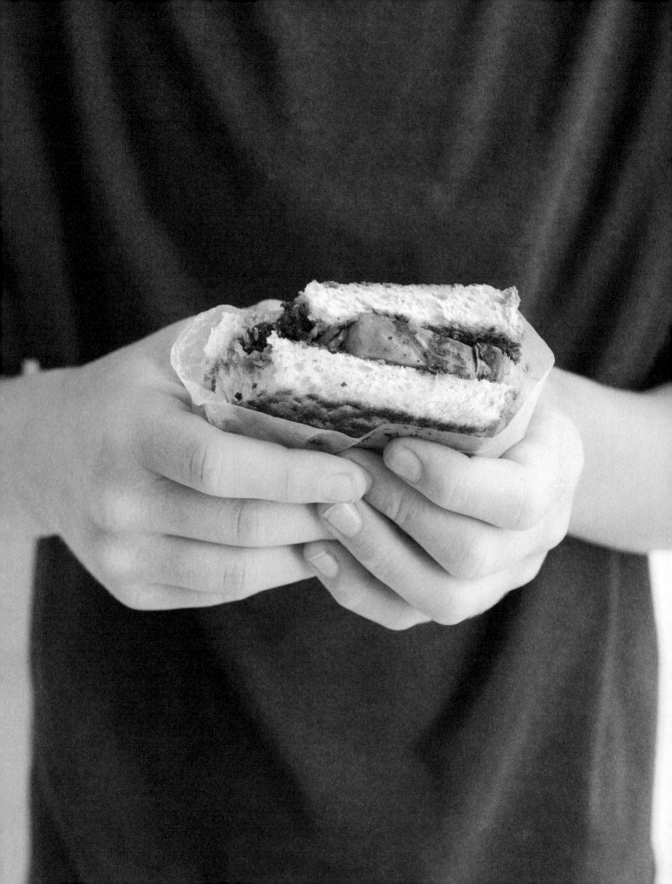

◀ Grilled Chicken and Pesto Sandwich

The combination of grilled chicken with fresh pesto works beautifully in this easy, yet savory grilled cheese sandwich. It takes leftover chicken to a whole new level!

Butter, for grilling

2 slices whole-grain bread

2 teaspoons (9 g) mayonnaise

2 teaspoons (10 g) Homemade Pesto (page 174)

2 ounces (40 g) cooked boneless chicken breast, sliced thin

1 slice (20 g) mozzarella cheese

Butter one side of both bread slices; flip over onto a cutting board.

Spread the mayonnaise and pesto on both bread slices. Layer the chicken and mozzarella, and close the sandwich.

Place the sandwich, buttered side down, on a skillet over medium heat. Grill for 2 to 3 minutes, until the cheese has begun to melt and the bread is golden brown. Press down with a spatula, flip, and grill the second side.

Remove from the pan onto a cutting board. Slice in half, and serve immediately or allow the sandwich to cool prior to packing in a lunchbox.

YIELD: 1 serving

Barbecue Chicken Sandwich

"Chicken isn't the same without barbecue sauce; it just tastes more plain," said my daughter one day. And just like that, this sandwich marked the end of plain chicken sandwiches for her.

4 ounces (113 g) oven roasted or grilled chicken, finely chopped

2 teaspoons (10 g) mayonnaise

2 teaspoons (10 g) barbecue sauce

Salt and pepper

2 slices whole-grain bread

Lettuce and tomato (optional)

In a bowl, combine the chicken, mayonnaise, and barbecue sauce. Season with the salt and pepper to taste.

Spread the chicken salad on one slice of bread. Dress the sandwich with lettuce and tomato (if your kids prefer it that way), and close the sandwich.

YIELD: 1 serving

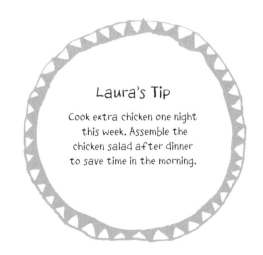

Laura's Tip

Cook extra chicken one night this week. Assemble the chicken salad after dinner to save time in the morning.

Grilled Chicken, Cheddar, and Grapes

The addition of juicy, fresh grapes not only brings a slight sweetness to this sandwich, but also helps to remoisten the leftover grilled chicken. The result is a delightful sandwich that kids and adults enjoy!

Butter, for grilling

2 slices whole-grain bread

2 teaspoons (9 g) mayonnaise

2 slices (40 g) medium Cheddar cheese, sliced thin

2 ounces (40 g) cooked chicken breast, thinly sliced

4 slivered red grapes

Butter one side of both bread slices; flip over onto a cutting board. Spread the mayonnaise on both slices of bread, and top with the cheese. Place the chicken over one slice, top with the grapes, and close the sandwich with the second cheese and bread slice.

Place the sandwich, buttered side down, on a skillet over medium heat. Grill for 2 to 3 minutes, until the cheese has begun to melt and the bread is golden brown. Press down with a spatula, flip, and grill the second side. Remove from the pan onto a cutting board.

Allow the grilled sandwich to cool for 5 minutes, and pack in a lunch container.

YIELD: 1 serving

Ricotta and Pesto Sandwich

This sandwich comes together easily with leftover pesto and ricotta from midweek dinners.

3 tablespoons (28 g) part-skim ricotta cheese

2 slices hearty oat bread, lightly toasted

1½ teaspoons Homemade Pesto (page 174)

Spread the ricotta onto one slice of bread, top with the pesto, and close the sandwich.

YIELD: 1 serving

Ninja Turtle Grilled Cheese

"Mom! I see green in my grilled cheese!" Well yes, Leonardo the Ninja Turtle gave me his recipe—enough said.

Butter, for grilling

2 slices sourdough bread

2 tablespoons (30 g) Homemade Pesto (page 174)

2 slices (40 g) mozzarella cheese

¼ avocado, sliced

2 tablespoons (19 g) goat cheese, crumbled

Small handful fresh baby spinach

Butter one side of each bread slice, and place buttered side down on a cutting board. Spread half of the pesto onto each slice of bread.

On one slice of the bread, add 1 slice of mozzarella cheese, the avocado, goat cheese, spinach, and the second slice of cheese, and then top it with the second slice of bread.

Place the sandwich in the pan, and grill for about 3 minutes, flip, and press down lightly. Cook for another 3 minutes until the second side is golden, and the cheese is melted.

YIELD: 1 serving

Grilled Leprechaun

You'll no longer throw away that one broccoli floret left over from dinner. From now on, you'll grill it and feel great that your kids are getting a little extra calcium, vitamin C, and iron in their lunch.

Butter, for grilling

2 slices whole-grain bread

2 slices (40 g) provolone cheese

1 broccoli floret, cooked and minced

Butter one side of both bread slices; flip over onto a cutting board. Place the cheese over both slices of bread. Spread the broccoli over one slice, and close the sandwich.

Place the sandwich, buttered side down, on a skillet over medium heat. Grill for 2 to 3 minutes, until the cheese has begun to melt and the bread is golden brown. Press down with a spatula, flip and grill the second side. Remove from the pan onto a cutting board.

Allow the grilled sandwich to cool down for 5 minutes before packing in a lunch container.

YIELD: 1 serving

Laura's Tip

Assemble this sandwich the night before, and grill in the morning. Wait a few minutes for the sandwich to cool down prior to packing it in a lunch container.

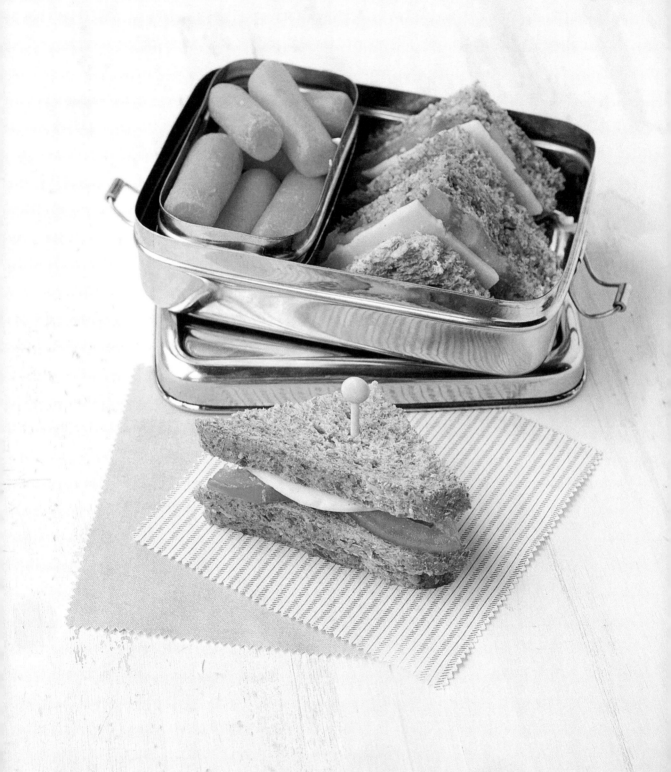

◀ Veggie Club

This veggie club is certain to convince you that a traditional club sandwich is overrated.

3 slices whole-wheat sandwich bread

2 tablespoons (30 g) Greek Hummus (page 175)

½ medium steak tomato, sliced thin

2 slices (40 g) provolone cheese

1 tablespoon (15 g) Homemade Pesto (page 174)

Lay all three bread slices on a cutting board. Spread half of the hummus onto one bread slice. Top with half of the tomato slices and one slice of cheese.

On the second slice of bread, spread half of the pesto and flip, pesto side down, to close the sandwich. Spread the remaining pesto on top of the second bread slice, and top with the remaining tomato slices and cheese. Spread the remaining hummus on the third bread slice and flip over to close the sandwich.

YIELD: 1 or 2 servings

Turkey and Hummus Sandwich

While I love this sandwich with all the fixings, my youngest prefers it plain and grilled. Either way, it's high in protein and full of flavor.

2 tablespoons (28 g) Greek Hummus (page 175)

2 slices whole-grain bread

2 slices (40 g) turkey

Lettuce leaves

Tomato slices

On a cutting board, spread the hummus on one slice of the bread, top with the turkey, lettuce, and tomato. Close the sandwich.

YIELD: 1 sandwich

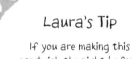

Laura's Tip

If you are making this sandwich the night before, place the turkey closest to the bread and the hummus in the middle. This will prevent the bread from getting soggy.

Apple Pie Sandwiches

Not exactly fresh out of the oven, but this sandwich has a certain "comfort food" taste that is second to none.

1 tablespoon (20 g) apple butter

1 tablespoon (16 g) almond or peanut butter

2 slices cinnamon raisin bread

Spread the apple butter and almond butter on the bread slices, and close the sandwich.

YIELD: 1 serving

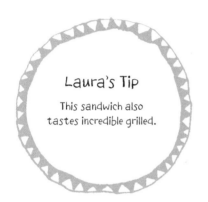

Laura's Tip

This sandwich also tastes incredible grilled.

Blueberry Heaven ▶

When I ran out of sandwich bread for lunch one day, I decided to use our favorite blueberry bread instead. Since then, I've ventured out and began using sweet breads in some of our lunches. When served with plenty of fresh fruit and veggies, it's not such a bad lunch after all.

1½ tablespoons (22 g) whipped cream cheese

2 slices Blueberry Bread (page 163)

Spread the cream cheese on both slices of bread. Close the sandwich.

YIELD: 1 serving

Sunny Side Sandwich

Sunshine and lemon bread are two things that make my son happy. The peanut butter and honey are just a bonus.

1½ tablespoons (8 g) peanut butter

2 slices Lemon Bread (page 164)

1 teaspoon honey

Carefully spread the peanut butter on one bread slice. Drizzle with the honey, and close the sandwich.

YIELD: 1 serving

Peaches and Cream Wafflewich ▶

Waffles make the perfect sandwich bread, especially when the filling is sweet and creamy!

2 tablespoons (30 g) cream cheese

2 Whole Wheat Waffles (page 44)

1 peach, sliced thin

Spread the cream cheese evenly on both waffles. Place the peach slices onto one of the waffles, and close the sandwich.

YIELD: 1 serving

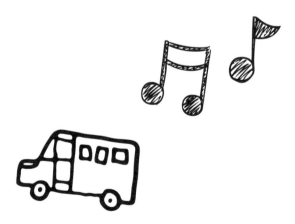

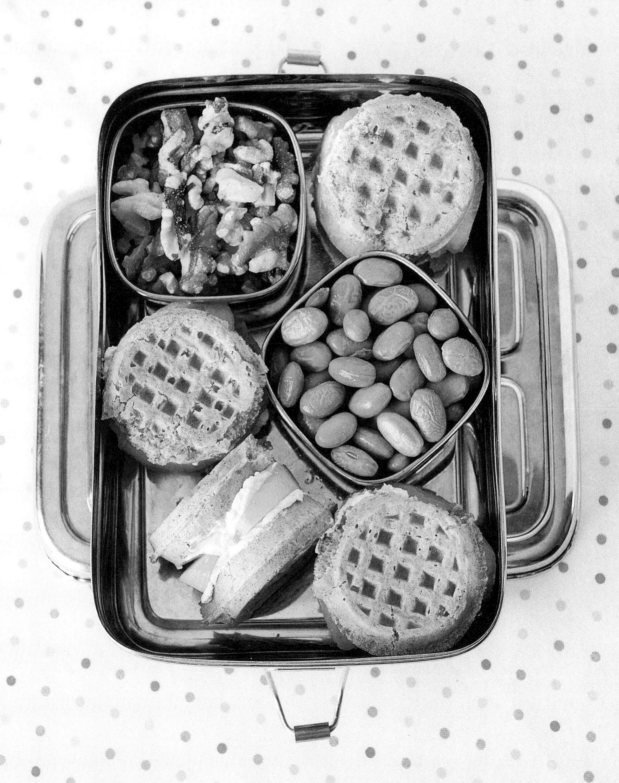

Strawberry Grilled Cheese

Sweet, sharp, and divine—this is one sandwich my daughter likes cut in triangles. Apparently, the smaller base prevents the strawberries from falling out. Kids …

Butter or oil, for grilling

2 slices sourdough bread

2 slices (40 g) white Cheddar cheese

¼ cup (45 g) fresh strawberries, thinly sliced

Butter one side of both bread slices; flip over onto a cutting board. On one of the slices, layer one slice of the cheese, the strawberries, and the remaining slice of cheese, and cover with the second slice of bread.

Place the sandwich, buttered side down, on a skillet over medium heat. Grill for 2 to 3 minutes, until the cheese has begun to melt and the bread is golden brown. Press down with a spatula, flip and grill the second side. Remove from the pan onto a cutting board.

Allow the grilled sandwich to cool for 5 minutes prior to packing in a lunch container.

YIELD: 1 serving

Strawberry Kiwi Wafflewich

Fresh, fruity, and the best way to "sandwich" kiwi. My son calls it a kiwi-wich.

4 tablespoons (60 g) cream cheese

4 Whole Wheat Waffles (page 44)

1 kiwifruit, peeled and sliced thin

2 or 3 strawberries, washed and sliced thin

Spread 1 tablespoon (15 g) cream cheese evenly on one side of all waffles. Layer the kiwi and strawberries onto two of the waffles. Top with the remaining waffles.

YIELD: 2 servings

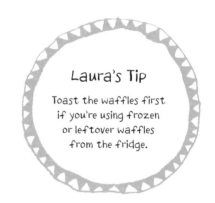

Laura's Tip

Toast the waffles first if you're using frozen or leftover waffles from the fridge.

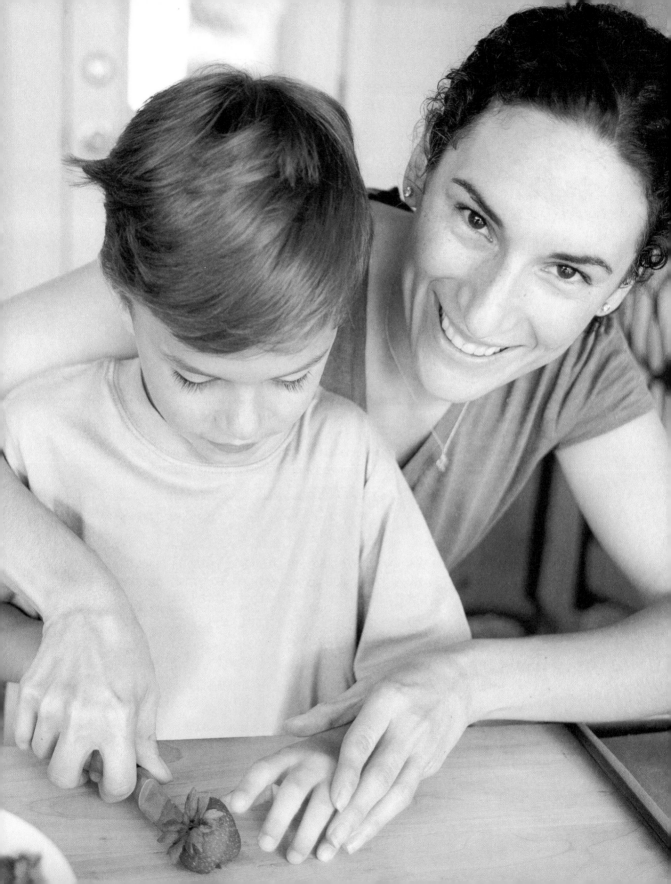

Lemon Sorbet Sandwich

This is another invention that resulted from one of those days where I ran out of sandwich bread. It's a little indulgent, so make sure you send lots of fruit and veggies with this one!

Two ½-inch (2.5 cm) slices Lemon Bread (page 164)

1½ tablespoons (23 g) whipped cream cheese

Lay the lemon bread on a cutting board. Spread the cream cheese over one slice, and close the sandwich.

YIELD: 1 serving

Dreamsicle Sandwich

All the creamy and delicious flavors of the classic frozen treat tucked away inside a whole-grain sandwich.

1½ tablespoons (23 g) cream cheese, softened

1 teaspoon frozen orange juice concentrate

2 slices whole-grain bread

½ teaspoon orange peel

In a small bowl, mix the cream cheese and juice concentrate until they are evenly combined. Spread the mixture on both slices of bread; then sprinkle orange peel on top. Close the sandwich.

YIELD: 1 serving

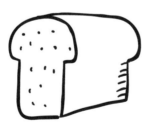

Berrylicious Sandwich

This sandwich is nothing short of amazing. One bite, and your kids will ask for it over and over again.

2 tablespoons (32 g) White Chocolate Peanut Butter (page 173)

2 slices whole-grain bread

¼ cup (35 g) raspberries

Spread the peanut butter on both slices of bread. Top with the raspberries, and close the sandwich.

YIELD: 1 serving

Roast Beef Farmer's Sandwich

Sometimes, you just need a satisfying meaty sandwich, and this one doesn't disappoint! As it turns out, I'm not the only one who loves this hearty roast beef favorite—my youngest devours it too!

1 tablespoon (15 g) plain Greek yogurt

½ teaspoon chopped fresh chives

Dash of garlic powder

Salt and pepper

2 slices whole wheat bread

2 or 3 slices (40 to 60 g) thinly sliced deli roast beef

¼ medium tomato, sliced

¼ cup (56 g) fresh arugula or baby spinach

In a small bowl, stir together the yogurt, chives, and garlic, and season with the salt and pepper to taste.

Spread the yogurt spread onto one slice of the bread, top with the roast beef, tomato, arugula, and remaining slice of bread.

YIELD: 1 serving

Kid's Philly Steak Sandwich

This simple, satisfying sandwich is the perfect kid-friendly version of the classic Philly Cheesesteak.

2 tablespoons (30 g) whipped cream cheese

2 slices whole-grain bread

2 slices (40 g) roast beef, sliced thin

Spread the cream cheese onto both slices of the bread. Top with the roast beef, and close the sandwich.

YIELD: 1 serving

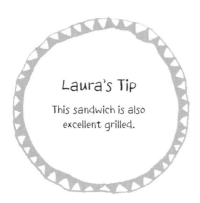

Laura's Tip

This sandwich is also excellent grilled.

Easy Muffuletta ▶

While the traditional muffuletta is made with a veggie olive salad, this version is easier to make and a lot more kid friendly.

One 10-inch (25.5 cm) round Italian bread

1 cup (160 g) Olive Salad (page 174)

Extra-virgin olive oil (optional)

4 ounces (80 g) Genoa salami

4 ounces (80 g) capicola or deli ham

3 or 4 thin slices mozzarella

3 or 4 thin slices provolone cheese

Cut the bread in half, lengthwise. Brush both cut sides with the oil from your olive salad, or the olive oil, if using, with more on the bottom half.

Begin layering the salami and ham on the bottom half of the bread. Top with the mozzarella and provolone cheese.

Next, add the olive salad from the center out. Place the other bread half on the top, and press it down without smashing the bread. Cut it into quarters.

For a school lunch: Wrap each quarter in parchment paper (or foil) to keep it together. Place inside a lunch bag.

YIELD: 4 servings

Kitchen Note

You can toast or warm up the sandwich in your oven for a few minutes prior to cutting. Alternatively, you can use a long Italian bread loaf if a round one is not available.

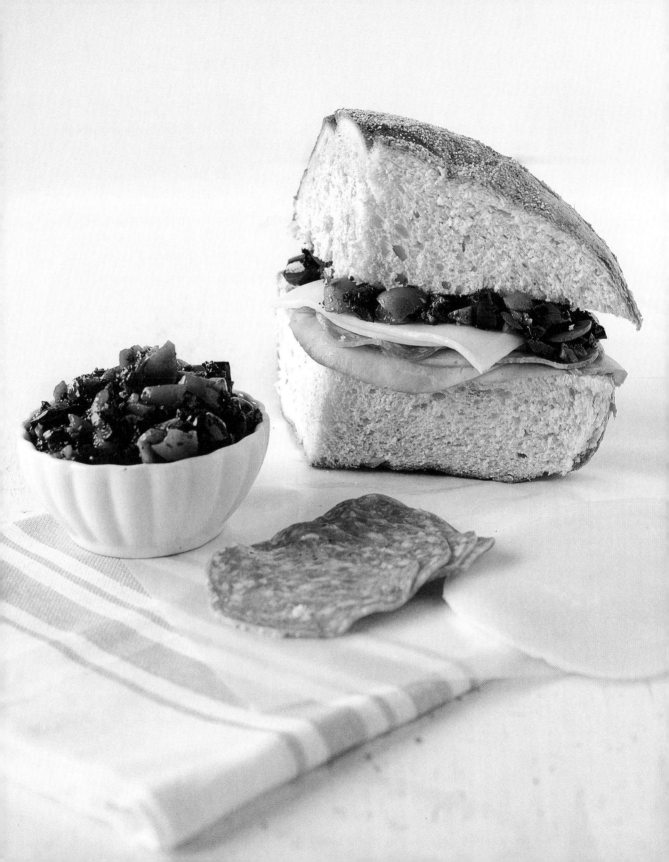

California Turkey Avocado Sandwich

In high school, we had a natural health food store across the street. They served the best turkey avocado sandwiches in town. To date, it's one of my favorite sandwich combinations.

2 teaspoons (9 g) mayonnaise

1 teaspoon mustard

2 slices whole-grain bread

2 slices (40 g) oven-baked turkey

1 slice (20 g) Swiss cheese

¼ avocado, thinly sliced

Small handful spinach leaves (optional)

¼ cup (65 g) Homemade Salsa (page 180)

In a small bowl, mix the mayonnaise and mustard.

On a cutting board, spread the mixture onto one side of both bread slices. Layer the turkey, cheese, and avocado. Top with the spinach leaves, if using, and close the sandwich.

Serve with fresh salsa on the side.

Optional: Grease or spray both outer sides of the sandwich, and grill over medium heat for about 3 minutes, press down on the sandwich, and grill the other side.

YIELD: 1 serving

Kitchen Note

Make this sandwich ahead of time, and store in the refrigerator. In the morning, grill it before packing it for school. Make sure you store the salsa in a small leak-proof container.

Grilled Meat Loaf Sandwich

This sandwich beats school cafeteria meat loaf any day! It's cheesy, delicious, and filling.

Butter, for grilling

2 slices whole-grain bread

⅓ cup (82 g) Veggie Tomato Sauce, (page 144), divided

2 slices (40 g) mozzarella cheese

1 slice leftover Veggie Meat Loaf (page 111)

Butter one side of both bread slices; flip over onto a cutting board. Spread about 1 tablespoon (15 g) tomato sauce thinly over both bread slices, top with the cheese, place the sliced meat loaf on top, and close the sandwich.

Place the sandwich, buttered side down, in a skillet over medium heat. Grill for 2 to 3 minutes, until the cheese has begun to melt and the bread is golden brown. Press down with a spatula, flip, and grill the second side. Remove from the pan onto a cutting board.

Allow the grilled sandwich to cool for 5 minutes before packing in a lunch container.

Serve with the remaining tomato sauce for dipping.

YIELD: 1 serving

Skinny Elvis

Sweet, salty, and a little bit crunchy, this sandwich will rock your kid's lunch world.

2 tablespoons (32 g) peanut butter

⅛ teaspoon cinnamon

2 slices whole-grain bread

¼ banana, sliced

1 teaspoon honey

2 slices (30 g) turkey bacon, cooked and crumbled

Spread the peanut butter on both slices of bread. Place the banana slices on top of the peanut butter on one slice of bread and sprinkle with cinnamon. Drizzle honey over the banana. Sprinkle the bacon on top of the banana, and close the sandwich.

Grilling is optional, but highly recommended by my daughter.

YIELD: 1 serving

The Elephant Sandwich

"Mom, this sandwich is going to make me big and strong and remember things." —Alex, age four.

2 tablespoons (32 g) peanut butter

2 slices whole-grain bread

½ banana, sliced or mashed

1 teaspoon honey

On a cutting board, spread peanut butter onto both bread slices. Top with the banana on one slice, drizzle honey over the banana, and close the sandwich.

YIELD: 1 serving

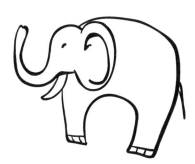

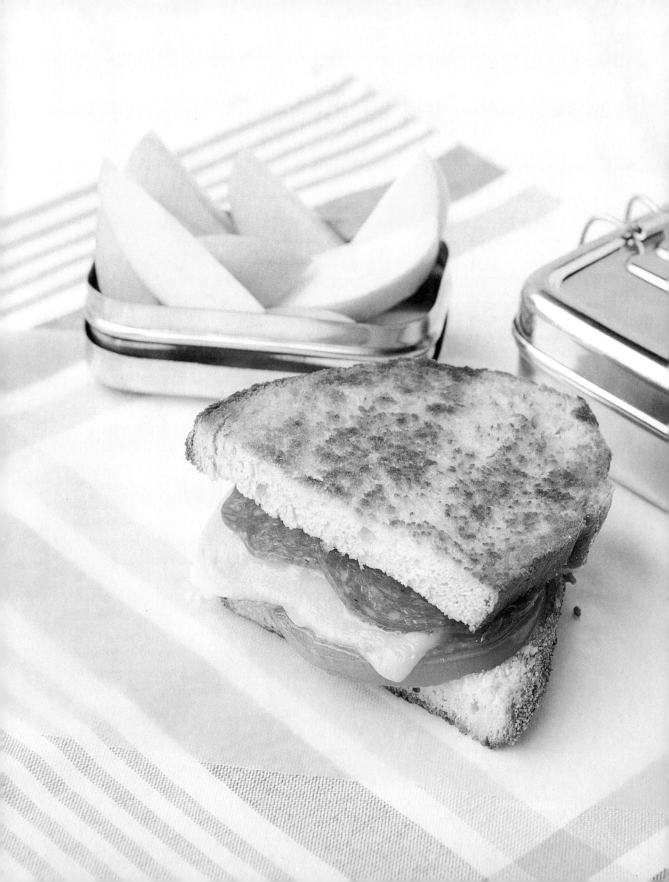

◀ Grilled Italian

While pregnant with my daughter, I traveled to Rome. On our seven-day trip, I devoured lots of grilled paninis. It's no wonder this is one of her favorite lunches.

Butter, for grilling

2 slices sourdough bread

1 tablespoon (14 g) mayonnaise

1 large slice tomato

2 slices (40 g) mozzarella cheese

5 thin slices (100 g) salami

Butter one side of both bread slices; flip over onto a cutting board. Spread mayonnaise onto one of the bread slices, layer the tomato, cheese, and salami, and close the sandwich.

Place the sandwich, buttered side down, in a skillet over medium heat. Grill for 2 to 3 minutes, until the cheese has begun to melt and the bread is golden brown. Press down with a spatula, flip, and grill the second side. Remove from the pan onto a cutting board.

Allow the grilled sandwich to cool for 5 minutes prior to packing in a lunch container.

YIELD: 1 serving

Swiss Tuna Melt

I never knew what tuna melts were until I met my Southern man. He could eat tuna like this every day for lunch. I must admit, his old habit is deliciously contagious.

1 can (6 ounces, or 170 g) water-packed tuna, drained

⅓ cup (37 g) shredded Swiss cheese

2 tablespoons (30 g) plain Greek yogurt or mayonnaise

¼ teaspoon black pepper

¼ teaspoon ground cumin

Butter, for grilling

4 slices whole-grain bread

In a large bowl, combine the tuna, cheese, yogurt, pepper, and cumin. Mix well until thoroughly combined.

Butter one side of both bread slices; flip over onto a cutting board. Divide the tuna mixture onto two slices of the bread, and top with the two additional slices of bread to close the sandwiches.

Place the sandwiches, buttered side down, on a skillet over medium heat. Grill for 2 to 3 minutes, until the cheese has begun to melt and the bread is golden brown. Press down with a spatula, flip, and grill the second side. Remove from the pan onto a cutting board. Allow the sandwiches to cool prior to slicing and packing inside a lunchbox.

YIELD: 2 servings

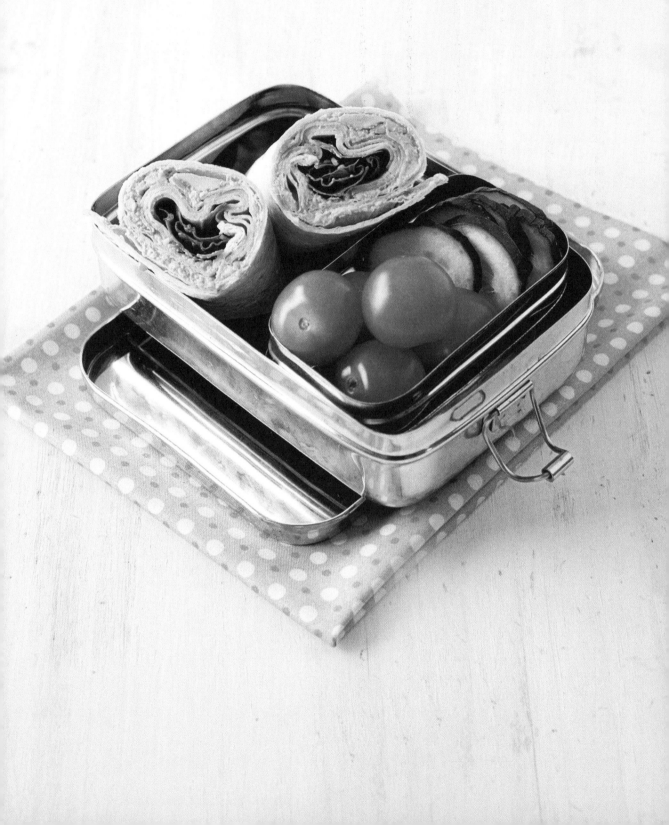

◀ Avocado Delight

One of my mottos: Cream cheese makes everything taste better. When I'm trying to introduce a new flavor or previously not-favored fruit, veggie, or protein to my kids, I often try the cream cheese route. I've since stopped stressing about my kids not eating things raw or not wanting to try an unfamiliar food. If it has cream cheese, they will, at the very least, try it.

¼ avocado, mashed

2 slices whole wheat bread or 1 wrap

1 tablespoon (15 g) whipped cream cheese

Salt and pepper

Spread the avocado on one slice of bread.

Spread the cream cheese on the other slice, season with the salt and pepper to taste, and close the sandwich.

YIELD: 1 serving

Hummus Monster

If ballparks served a healthy sandwich, I think this would be it. It has all the classic pretzel and mustard flavors, but added nutrition thanks to the veggies and hummus.

1 round pretzel roll

1 teaspoon mustard

1 tablespoon (15 g) hummus

1 or 2 thin tomato slices

1 or 2 lettuce leaves

On a cutting board, slice the roll in half. Spread the mustard thinly over both halves, and top with the hummus.

Layer the tomato and lettuce on one of the slices, and close the roll.

YIELD: 1 serving

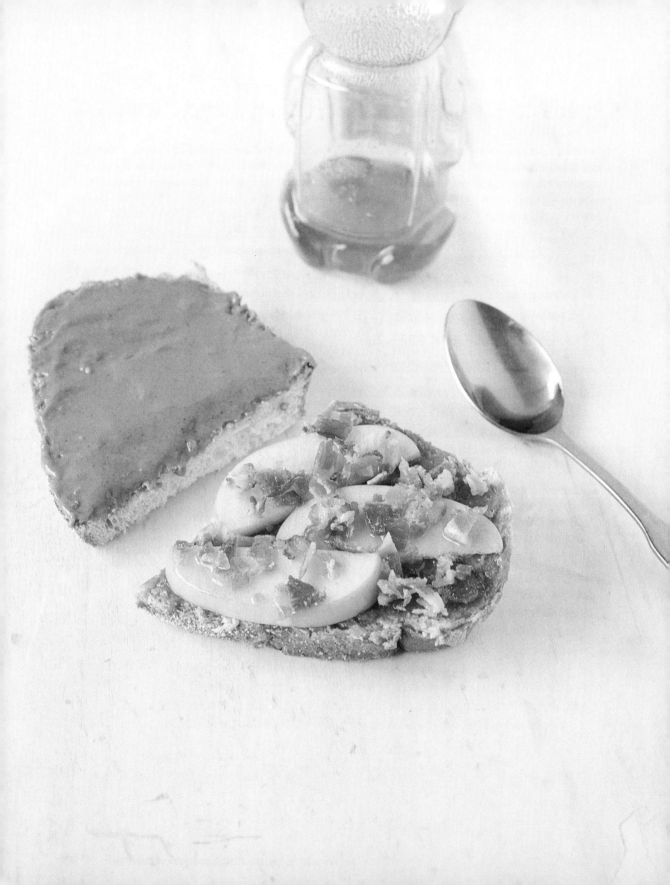

The Nathan

My friend Rachel's husband, Nathan, says this sandwich has all his favorite things from childhood mixed in. My kids and I were skeptical, but once we tried it, we loved it!

2 tablespoons (32 g) peanut butter

2 slices whole-grain bread

¼ Granny Smith apple, sliced thin

1 teaspoon honey

1 strip bacon (15 g), cooked and crumbled

On a cutting board, spread peanut butter on both bread slices. On one bread slice, distribute apple on top of the peanut butter. Drizzle honey on top of the apple. Sprinkle crumbled bacon over the apple. Close the sandwich.

YIELD: 1 serving

Ham and Cheese "Waffle"

Is it a waffle? Is it a ham and cheese sandwich? It's both!

1 batch Whole Wheat Waffle batter (page 44)

½ cup (75 g) chopped deli ham

¾ cup (90 g) shredded mozzarella cheese

1 teaspoon dried basil

½ teaspoon dried oregano

Preheat the waffle maker.

After preparing the waffle batter, add the ham, cheese, basil, and oregano to the batter. With a spatula, fold to combine the ingredients.

Spoon ⅓ to ½ cup (150 to 180 g) batter onto the hot waffle maker (this will vary by the size of your waffle maker). Spread the batter to within ¼ inch of the edge of the grids. Close the lid, and bake until the waffle is golden brown.

YIELD: 4 to 6 waffles

Kitchen Note

Make the waffles ahead of time. Store in the refrigerator or freeze. In the morning, toast thoroughly, and pack in a stainless steel lunch container. Pair them with our Tomato Veggie Soup (page 150).

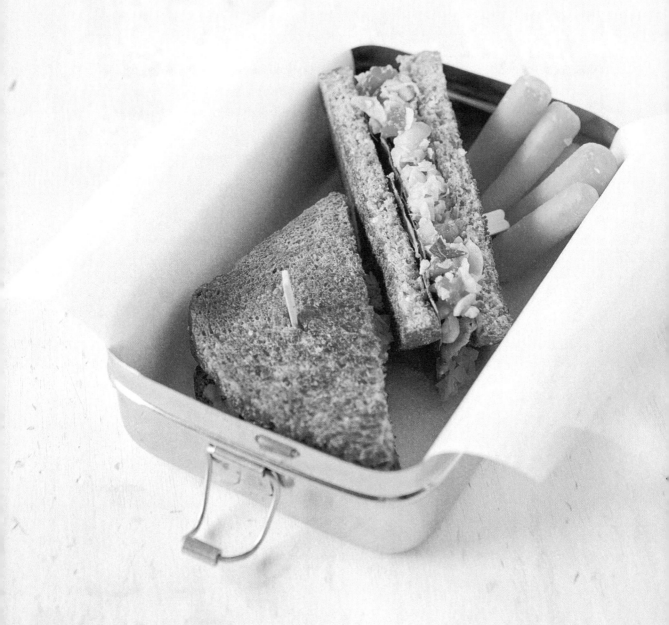

Mashed Chickpea Sandwich

This flavorful spread is perfect for making a quick sandwich, or packing as a dip for your favorite whole-grain crackers.

1 can (15 ounces, or 450 g) chickpeas, rinsed and drained

2 tablespoons (30 ml) lemon juice

1½ tablespoons (23 ml) extra-virgin olive oil

2 tablespoons (23 g) roasted red bell pepper, chopped

1 tablespoon (10 g) finely chopped red onion

2 tablespoons (8 g) fresh parsley, chopped

Salt and pepper

4 slices whole-grain bread

Handful of fresh spinach, (optional)

In a medium bowl, using a fork, mash half of the chickpeas. Add in the remaining chickpeas, lemon juice, olive oil, bell pepper, onion, and parsley. Season with the salt and pepper to taste.

Spoon the mixture onto two slices of the bread, add spinach, if using, and close the sandwiches with the remaining slices of bread. Or eat it straight from the bowl with a few whole-grain crackers.

YIELD: 2 servings

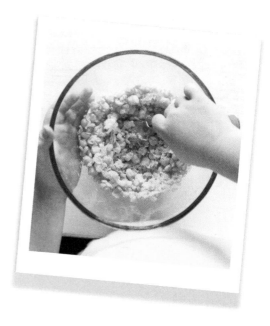

Pure Pastrami

A sandwich made for simple kids, such as my daughter, who loves the salty cured flavor of pastrami.

1 teaspoon mustard

2 teaspoons (9 g) mayonnaise

2 slices whole-grain bread

4 thin slices (80 g) pastrami

Combine the mustard and mayonnaise in a small bowl.

Place the bread on a cutting board. Spread the mayonnaise mixture onto both slices. Layer the pastrami on one of the slices, and close the sandwich.

YIELD: 1 serving

Hawaiian Sliders ▶

Bite-size, sweet, and delicious. These are a kid favorite!

1 teaspoon yellow mustard

2 teaspoons (9 g) mayonnaise

2 Hawaiian rolls

2 slices (40 g) ham

2 pineapple rings

In a small bowl, combine the mustard and mayonnaise. Slice the rolls in half, and spread the mustard and mayonnaise thinly over each roll.

Cut the ham slices in half, then fold each half into quarters. Place a folded ham quarter over each roll half, top two of those with a pineapple ring, and top with other roll half to close the rolls.

YIELD: 1 serving

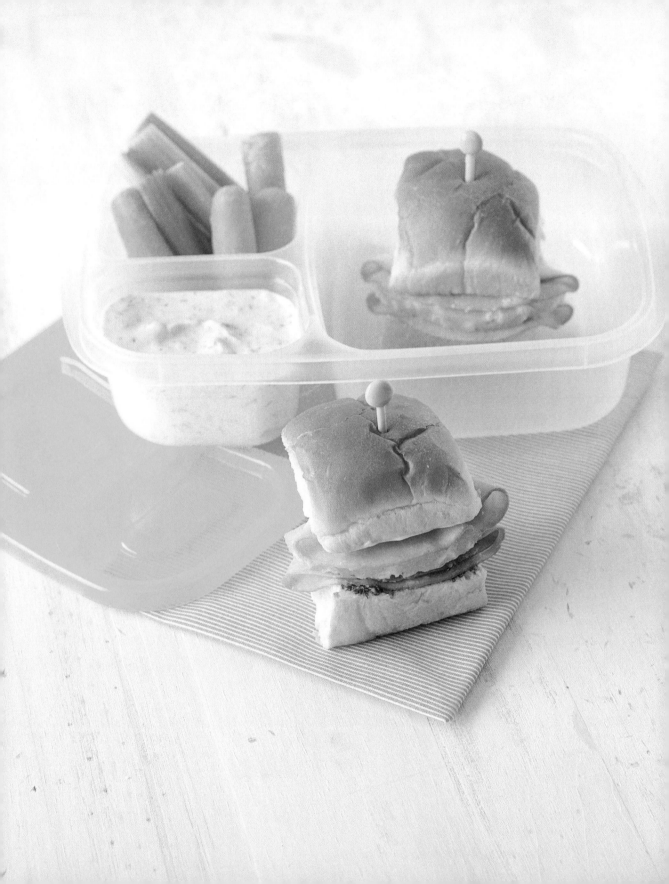

Chicken Salad Sliders

You'd better watch out when you make these chicken salad sliders! If you leave them unattended while making lunch, you may come back and notice that you are missing one or two. Yes, they are that good!

1 whole roasted chicken, meat removed

3 tablespoons (18 g) lemon juice

½ cup (115 g) mayonnaise

¼ teaspoon salt

½ teaspoon black pepper

1 teaspoon ground cumin

½ cup (60 g) finely chopped celery

12 Hawaiian sweet rolls

Put the cooked chicken in a food processor, and pulse a few times to roughly chop. Stir, then continue pulsing for another 15 to 30 seconds, until the chicken is finely chopped. (Note: If you turn on the food processor and let it go, your chicken will become a paste instead of finely chopped. So be sure to pulse the chicken for best results.)

In a large bowl, combine the lemon juice, mayonnaise, salt, pepper, and cumin, and blend until thoroughly combined. Add the chicken to the mayo mixture, and fold with a spatula. Next, fold in the celery.

Slice the rolls in half horizontally. Top each roll bottom half with a few tablespoons of the chicken salad. Close with the top of the roll.

YIELD: 6 servings

Cucumber Goat Cheese Sliders

Cucumber sandwiches are a classic finger food. This unique version pairs whipped cream cheese with goat cheese for a tangy undertone that complements the sweetness of the Hawaiian rolls.

1 tablespoon (15 g) whipped cream cheese

1 tablespoon (15 g) goat cheese

2 sweet Hawaiian rolls

¼ cucumber, thinly sliced

In a small bowl, mix the cream cheese and goat cheese until creamy and well combined.

Cut the rolls in half, then divide the cheese mixture evenly over both sides of the rolls, place the cucumber on one side, and close the sliders.

YIELD: 2 sliders

Caprese Sliders

What's better than fresh tomatoes, basil, and mozzarella? Sandwiching the fresh flavors in soft, sweet Hawaiian bread, of course!

2 Hawaiian dinner rolls, sliced in half

1 tablespoon (30 g) Homemade Pesto (page 174)

2 thick tomato slices

2 thick slices of fresh mozzarella

Open the Hawaiian rolls and thinly spread the pesto sauce over both halves.

Place the tomatoes on the bottom half of the rolls, top with the mozzarella, and close the sliders.

YIELD: 1 serving

Norwegian Tea Sandwich

In Spain, my grandmother would make these sandwiches for birthday parties, appetizers, or a special occasion. I loved the combination of the salty smoked salmon and sweet cream cheese. Happily, so do my kids.

1½ tablespoons (19 g) whipped cream cheese

2 slices soft sandwich bread

2 ounces (57 g) smoked salmon

Spread the cream cheese onto both bread slices, place the salmon on top of one slice, and close the sandwich.

YIELD: 1 serving

Laura's Tip

On hot days, consider putting the sandwich in the freezer the night before. In the morning, cut and pack it in a lunchbox. They will be the perfect temperature for lunch, and you won't need ice packs.

PB & J Pinwheels ▶

This recipe takes the classic peanut butter and jelly for a spin.

2 whole-wheat bread slices

2 tablespoons (32 g) peanut butter

1 tablespoon (20 g) jelly

Using a serrated knife, cut the crusts from the whole wheat bread slices. Flatten each slice with a rolling pin.

Spread the peanut butter and jelly on the prepared bread slices and roll tightly. Cut each roll in half and then into 1-inch (2.5 cm) pieces.

YIELD: 1 serving

Strawberry Fruit Leather ▶

Who knew making fruit leather could be this simple? Feel free to experiment with your child's favorite fruit.

5 cups (850 g) strawberries, hulled and halved

2 tablespoons (42 g) honey

Preheat the oven to the lowest temperature setting, which will probably be somewhere in between 150°F and 200°F (65°C and 93°C).

In a medium saucepan over low heat, cook the strawberries until they are soft and the juices begin to release. Add the honey and stir until combined.

Pour into a food processor or blender and purée. If your kids don't like the seeds, pour the mixture through a fine-mesh strainer.

Line a baking sheet with parchment paper, and pour the berry mixture onto the sheet. Bake for 4 to 6 hours, until the fruit leather peels away easily from the parchment. Once cooled, cut the fruit leather (with parchment) into strips.

YIELD: 12 to 14 strips

Kitchen Note

Don't pour too thin of a layer, or you'll have fruit crisps instead of fruit leather. If it's too thick, it will take longer to dehydrate. An even consistent layer in both color and thickness works best.

All oven temperatures vary, so begin checking after 3½ hours of baking, and remember: The center of the tray always takes longer than the edges.

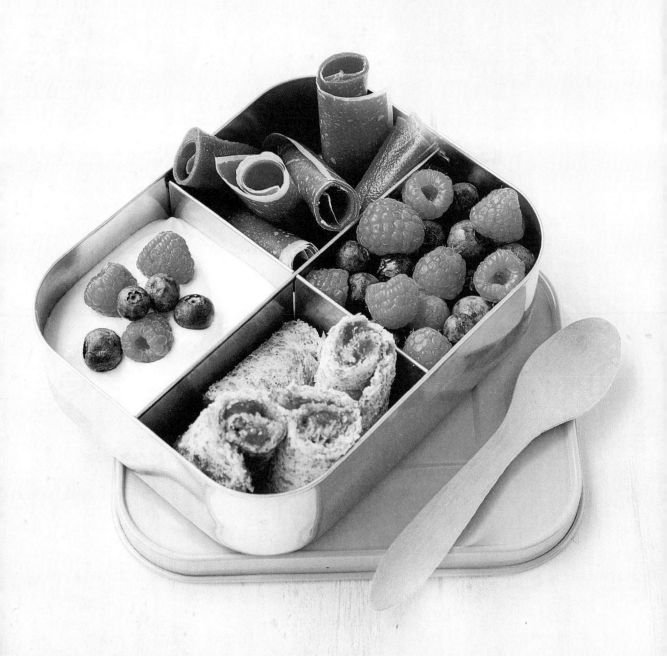

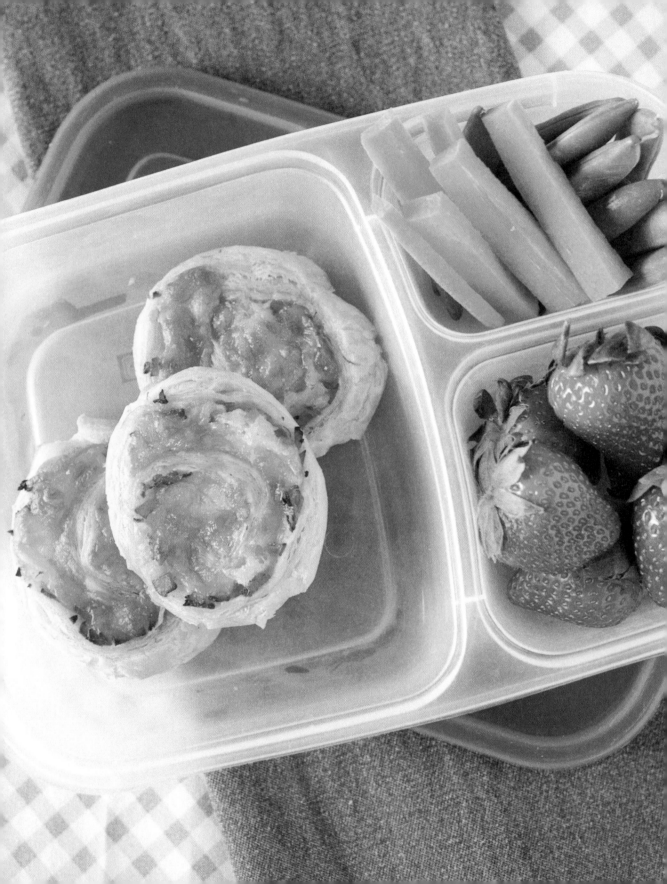

◀ Hawaiian Puff-Wheels

My daughter loves finding these in her lunchbox. She says they are fancy and delicious. The variations are endless, so this one recipe can yield many happy lunchboxes for years to come.

1 package (17 ounces, or 490 g) puff pastry sheets, thawed

¾ cup (112 g) sliced deli ham, finely chopped

½ cup (80 g) crushed pineapple, well drained

1¼ cups (145 g) shredded Cheddar cheese

Preheat the oven to 375°F (190°C), and line a baking sheet with parchment paper.

On a lightly floured surface, unroll the pastry sheets. Spread the ham and pineapple evenly over both sheets. Sprinkle with the cheese.

Carefully roll the dough, starting with the long side so that you end up with a long log. Cut the filled dough into 1-inch (2.5 cm) thick pieces, and place on the baking sheet.

Bake for 10 to 12 minutes until the dough rises and is golden. Remove from the oven, and allow the wheels to cool for 5 minutes prior to packing in a lunchbox. If you make these the night before, pack them chilled in the lunchbox. They will be room temperature by lunch.

YIELD: 4 or 5 servings

Recipe Variations

- ½ cup (80 g) crumbled bacon + 1¼ cups (150 g) Cheddar cheese

- ¼ cup (65 g) pesto sauce + ½ cup (75 g) crumbled feta + ½ cup (60 g) mozzarella cheese

---

Cuban Pinwheels

Craving a Cuban sandwich, but realizing we were out of bread, I resorted to my favorite go-to option—flour tortillas! This Cuban sandwich wrap is now a staple in our lunch rotation—it's fast, easy, and delicious!

One 8-inch (20 cm) tortilla

2 slices (40 g) honey ham

2 slices (40 g) pastrami

2 slices (40 g) provolone cheese

Layer the tortilla with the ham, pastrami, and cheese. Roll tightly. Cut the tortilla roll in half, and then into 1-inch (2.5 cm) rounds.

Optional: After layering the ingredients, transfer the tortilla into a skillet. Grill the tortilla open-faced for about 3 minutes on medium-low heat, remove from the pan, and roll.

YIELD: 1 serving

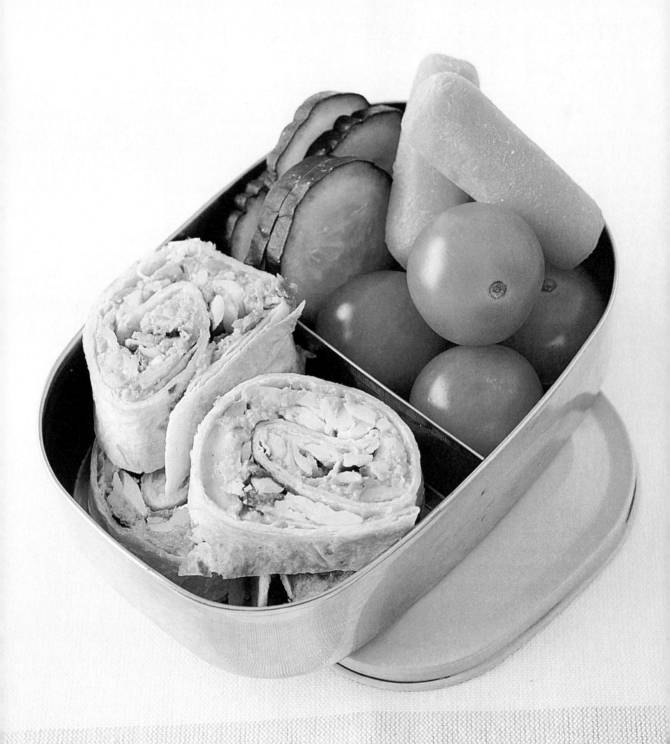

◀ ABC Pinwheels

I love the combination of avocado and bacon. The sweet flavor of ripe avocado paired with the crunchy, salty flavor of bacon is definitely worth each savory bite.

¼ avocado, mashed

2 teaspoons (10 g) mayonnaise

One 8-inch (20 cm) flour tortilla

2 slices (15 g) bacon, cooked and crumbled

2 tablespoons (15 g) shredded, white Cheddar cheese

In a small bowl, mash the avocado and mix with the mayonnaise.

Place the tortilla on a cutting board, and spread the mayonnaise–avocado mixture evenly over the top. Top with the bacon and cheese.

Roll the tortilla tightly. Cut the tortilla roll in half, and then into 1-inch (2.5 cm) pieces.

YIELD: 1 serving

Tapenade Pinwheels

My daughter, the olive lover, often asks for extra olives on the side. Some weeks, she asks for this lunch twice.

One 8-inch (20 cm) flour tortilla

2 tablespoons (13 g) whipped cream cheese

¼ cup (25 g) Olive Salad (page 174)

Place the tortilla on a cutting board and spread the cream cheese evenly over the tortilla. Top with the olive salad.

Roll the tortilla tightly. Cut the tortilla roll in half, and then into 1-inch (2.5 cm) pieces.

YIELD: 1 serving

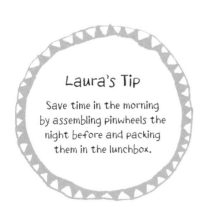

Laura's Tip

Save time in the morning by assembling pinwheels the night before and packing them in the lunchbox.

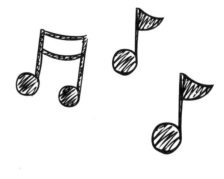

Pesto Swirls

Swirls are a fun alternative to pizza. Enjoyed warm, or at room temperature, they are perfect for on-the-go lunches.

1 Pizza Dough (page 167)

½ cup (130 g) prepared pesto

¼ cup (25 g) grated Parmesan cheese + additional for topping (optional)

Prepare the pizza dough according to the recipe directions.

After the dough rises, roll it out onto a greased surface, silicone mat, or parchment paper. Roll it into an 18 × 10-inch (45.7 × 25.4 cm) rectangle. Spread the presto sauce onto the dough and sprinkle on the cheese, leaving 1 inch (2.5 cm) free of sauce along the top edge.

Beginning with the edge closest to you, roll the dough into a log, pinching the seam closed. Cut the log into 12 slices. Place the rolls on a parchment-lined baking sheet.

Cover and let rise for about 1 hour, or until puffy. Sprinkle with additional cheese, if using. Toward the end of the rising time, preheat the oven to 350°F (180°C).

Bake for 20 to 24 minutes or until golden brown. Remove the rolls from the oven, and serve immediately. Refrigerate leftovers, and in the morning, pack the rolls in a lunchbox to be enjoyed at room temperature.

YIELD: 12 rolls

Kitchen Note

If using prepared dough, roll out the dough and prepare according to the recipe. Bake according to the package instructions, checking the rolls 5 minutes before the pizza time on package.

All ovens vary, and so does prepared pizza dough, so check for a golden brown color around your edges.

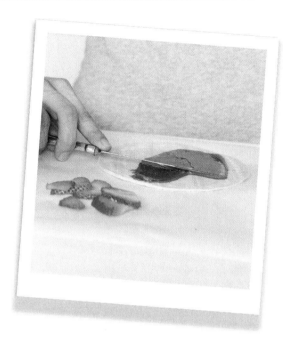

Chocolate Flautas

One weekend morning, I wanted to make chocolate crepes for my kids, but I had no eggs! Since the kids already had their mind set on crepes for breakfast, I substituted with whole-grain tortillas instead. The kids loved them, and they've since become a lunchbox favorite as well.

One 8-inch (20 cm) whole-grain flour tortilla

2 tablespoons (32 g) Easy Homemade Chocolate Spread (page 171)

½ cup (85 g) strawberries, sliced

Lay the tortilla on a cutting board. Distribute the chocolate spread over the tortilla.

Beginning at one end, roll tightly. Cut the roll in half and secure with a bento pick or lunch skewer. Serve with the strawberries.

YIELD: 1 serving

Honey Mustard Chicken Wrap

This wrap is hearty and filling and combines the great flavors of honey mustard and chicken, which kids love.

1 tablespoon (11 g) honey mustard

One 8-inch (20 cm) tortilla

2 slices (40 g) deli roasted chicken, or 2 ounces (40 g) cooked chicken, chopped

1 slice (20 g) Cheddar cheese

1 leaf green-leaf lettuce

¼ medium tomato, diced

On a cutting board, spread the honey mustard over the tortilla, leaving a ½-inch (1.3 cm) rim all the way around.

Top the tortilla with the chicken, cheese, lettuce, and tomato. Roll tightly and cut in half.

YIELD: 1 serving

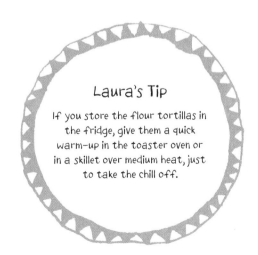

Laura's Tip

If you store the flour tortillas in the fridge, give them a quick warm-up in the toaster oven or in a skillet over medium heat, just to take the chill off.

Crunchy Carrot Wrap

My daughter will only eat veggies when they are crunchy, which is a good thing because they are most nutritous that way. The addition of honey and ricotta adds a creamy sweetness that makes raw veggies irresistible for kids and adults alike!

One 8-inch (20 cm) tortilla

2 tablespoons (30 g) ricotta cheese

¼ cup (28 g) carrots, finely shredded

2 teaspoons (14 g) honey

½ teaspoon grated lemon peel

Lay the tortilla on a cutting board. Spread the ricotta over the tortilla, leaving a ½-inch (1.3 cm) rim at the edges. Layer the carrots evenly. Drizzle with the honey and top with the lemon peel. Roll tightly, and cut the wrap in half.

YIELD: 1 serving

Little Italy Wrap

It's like a pizza, but wrapped—and fast!

One 8-inch (20 cm) tortilla

5 thin slices (100 g) salami

2 slices (40 g) mozzarella cheese

1 Roma tomato, finely diced

Lay the tortilla on a cutting board. Layer the salami and cheese evenly. Top with the tomato. Roll tightly, and cut the wrap in half.

YIELD: 1 serving

All My Veggies Wrap

It can be hard to get kids to eat salad, but in this wrap, they won't even notice they are eating lots of veggies! The pesto also provides a boost of nutrition.

1 tablespoon (15 g) Homemade Pesto (page 174)

One 8-inch (20 cm) tortilla

2 or 3 butterhead lettuce leaves

¼ cup (28 g) carrots, shredded

¼ cucumber, julienned

On a cutting board, spread the pesto over the tortilla. Layer the lettuce leaves, and top with the carrots and cucumber. Roll tightly and cut in half.

YIELD: 1 serving

Turkey Avocado Wrap

When in doubt: wrap, pack, and serve.

One 8-inch (20 cm) spinach wrap

1 tablespoon (15 g) plain Greek yogurt

¼ teaspoon Arriba! Seasoning (page 106)

¼ avocado, diced

3 slices (60 g) oven roasted turkey

¼ cup (65 g) Homemade Salsa (page 180)

Lay the wrap on a cutting board and spread with the yogurt. Sprinkle with the seasoning, then layer the avocado and turkey.

Roll tightly and cut in half. Pack the salsa in a small container with a lid.

YIELD: 1 serving

Pizza Man Wheels

Similar to the pesto swirls, but for kids who would rather eat more traditional pizza with tomato sauce.

1 Pizza Dough (page 167)

½ cup (125 g) pizza sauce or Veggie Tomato Sauce (page 144)

¼ cup (25 g) grated Parmesan cheese + additional for sprinkling (optional)

½ cup (38 g) grated mozzarella cheese

Prepare the pizza dough according to the recipe directions.

After the dough rises, roll it out onto a greased surface, silicone mat, or parchment paper. Roll it into an 18 × 10-inch (45.7 × 25 cm) rectangle. Spread the sauce onto the dough and sprinkle on the cheeses, leaving 1 inch (2.5 cm) free of sauce along the top edge.

Beginning with the edge closest to you, roll the dough into a log, pinching the seam closed. Cut the log into 12 slices.

Place rolls on a parchment-lined baking sheet. Cover and let rise for about 1 hour, or until puffy. Sprinkle with additional Parmesan cheese, if using. Toward the end of the rising time, preheat the oven to 350°F (180°C).

Bake for 20 to 24 minutes or until golden brown. Remove the rolls from the oven, and serve immediately.

For a school lunch: Pack the rolls in a lunchbox to be enjoyed at room temperature.

YIELD: 12 rolls

Kitchen Note

If using prepared dough, roll out the dough, spread the ingredients evenly, and bake according to package instructions, checking the rolls 5 minutes before the pizza time on the package.

All ovens vary and so do prepared pizza rolls. Check for a golden brown color around your edges to ensure proper doneness.

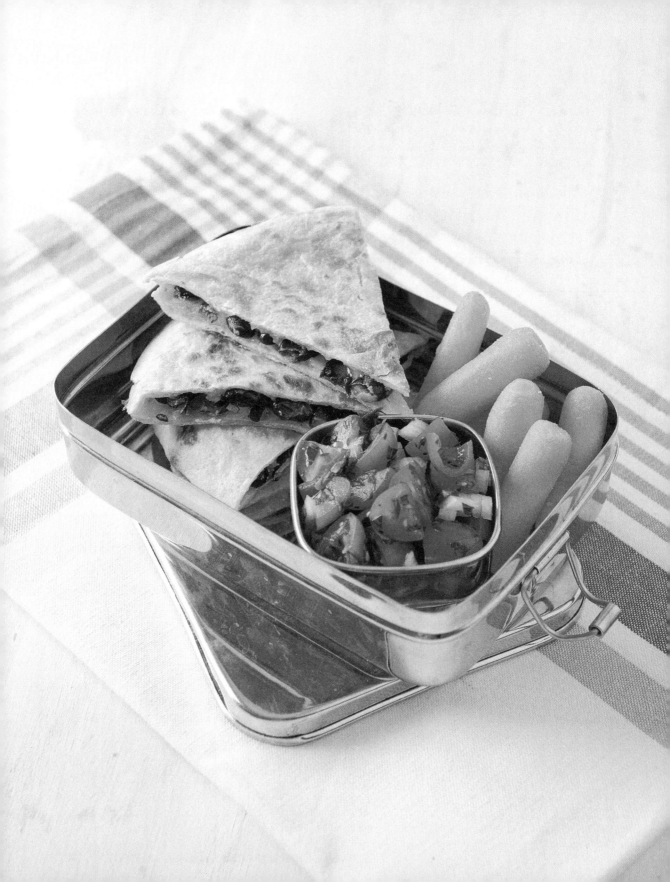

Black Bean Quesadillas

It's a myth that quesadillas need to be hot and the cheese needs to be gooey and melty for kids to love them. They are excellent at room temperature and the perfect disguise for healthy things—such as beans.

¼ cup (25 g) canned black beans, rinsed

2 tablespoons (16 g) frozen corn, thawed

1 tablespoon (9 g) scallions, chopped very small (optional)

2 teaspoons (1 g) fresh cilantro, chopped

1 teaspoon Arriba! Seasoning (page 106)

¼ cup (30 g) shredded Cheddar cheese

Two 8-inch (20 cm) tortillas

2 ounces (55 g) Homemade Salsa (page 180)

In a large bowl, place the beans, corn, onion, if using, cilantro, seasoning, and cheese. Gently mix until everything is evenly combined.

Scoop the filling and place on top of one side of one tortilla. Top with the second tortilla.

In a warm skillet, cook both sides over medium heat until the tortilla is brown and crispy, and the cheese has melted.

For a school lunch: I like to assemble quesadillas the night before. In the morning, I slowly grill them while I pour myself a cup of coffee. After the quesadilla is grilled, I lay it on a cutting board to cool, usually while I am getting the kids dressed. Then, simply cut and pack them inside the lunchbox.

YIELD: 1 or 2 servings

Kitchen Note

Why not make extra quesadillas and freeze them? Assemble quesadillas and place flat on a cookie sheet lined with parchment paper. Once the quesadillas are flash frozen, about 1 hour, transfer to a freezer bag and store flat.

To reheat: Warm in the microwave, or grill in a skillet on low, so you won't burn the tortilla and all the ingredients have time to warm and the cheese to melt.

Pizza Dough Stromboli

The debate is out there about where to get the best stromboli in any given city. For my family, however, the best comes straight out of my oven.

1 Pizza Dough (page 167)

1 cup (150 g) mozzarella cheese, grated and divided

¼ cup (25 g) grated Parmesan cheese + additional for topping

½ cup (125 g) pizza sauce or Veggie Tomato Sauce (page 144) + additional for dipping

¼ pound (60 g) Genoa salami

¼ pound (60 g) honey ham

1 egg, beaten

Make the pizza dough following the recipe directions.

Preheat the oven to 500°F (250°C). Line a baking sheet with parchment paper, and set aside.

In a small bowl, combine the cheeses. Roll out the pizza dough onto the baking sheet to approximately 10 × 16 inches (25 × 40.6 cm). Spread the sauce over two-thirds of the dough lengthwise, leaving about 3 inches (7.5 cm) of plain dough along one of the edges.

Top the sauce with half of the cheese mix, then the salami and ham, and then the remaining cheese mix.

Brush the plain strip of dough with the egg. Roll up into a log, lengthwise, starting with the end filled with toppings and ending with the plain strip of dough at the bottom of the roll. Pinch the ends or tuck them in.

Lightly coat the entire stromboli with egg. Cut slats on the top of the dough every 2 inches (5 cm), so that steam can escape. Sprinkle with the additional Parmesan cheese, and bake for 12 to 14 minutes or until golden brown.

Allow the stromboli to cool for 5 minutes before slicing into pieces. Serve with the additional sauce.

For a school lunch: In the morning, lightly warm up a piece of stromboli in a toaster oven or regular oven. Store pizza sauce in a small leak-proof container, and pack in the lunchbox. Stromboli is great at room temperature.

YIELD: 4 to 6 servings

Pizza Dippers

My friend, Kendra Peterson, has a way of repurposing leftovers so that they don't look the same as the original dish. She took pizza slices and created the dippers.

2 slices leftover pizza

¼ cup (62 g) Veggie Tomato Sauce (page 144)

Cut leftover pizza into thin strips. Serve with the tomato sauce.

YIELD: 1 serving

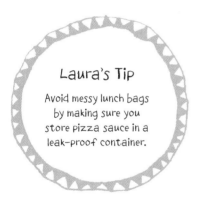

Laura's Tip

Avoid messy lunch bags by making sure you store pizza sauce in a leak-proof container.

Green Eggs and Ham Pizza

Your family will beg for that single leftover slice; so you might as well double the recipe and make more for everyone. That way, you have something to pack for lunch!

1 Pizza Dough (page 167)

1 cup (245 g) pizza sauce or Veggie Tomato Sauce (page 144)

2½ cups (290 g) shredded mozzarella cheese

4 hard-boiled eggs, chopped

8 ounces (160 g) sliced honey ham, chopped

½ cup (50 g) green olives, sliced

Prepare the pizza dough, following the recipe directions, and preheat the oven to 375°F (190°C).

Using a rolling pin, roll out one of the dough balls onto a floured surface. Transfer it to a floured baking sheet.

Spread half of the pizza sauce on to the base, leaving a ½-inch (1.3 cm) border all the way around. Layer half of the cheese over the sauce and begin to distribute half of the toppings evenly: eggs, ham, and olives. Repeat the process with the second dough ball and the remaining ingredients.

Bake the pizzas in the oven for about 22 to 25 minutes, until the edges are golden and have risen. Remove from the oven.

YIELD: 6 servings

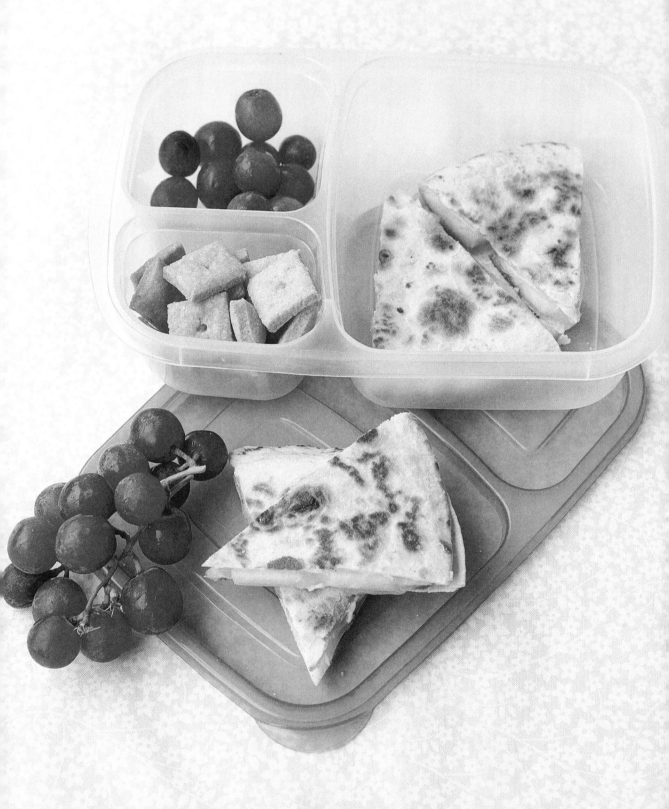

Cheddar and Pear Quesadillas

This creative quesadilla inspired my daughter to enjoy pears. The tangy sharp Cheddar cheese paired with sweet ripe pears creates a wonderful flavor combination that kids of all ages enjoy!

1 tablespoon (14 g) mayonnaise

2 teaspoons (8 g) mustard

Two 8-inch (20 cm) flour tortillas

1 small pear, sliced thin

⅓ cup (38 g) shredded sharp Cheddar cheese

Oil for grilling

In a small dish, mix the mayonnaise and mustard.

Spread a thin layer of the mayo–mustard spread over each tortilla. Spread the pear over one tortilla, sprinkle the cheese over the pear, and then top with the second tortilla, mayo-mustard side down.

Brush the bottom side of the tortilla with oil, and grill in a 10-inch (25 cm) skillet over medium heat until the cheese is melted, about 2 to 3 minutes. Brush the top of the tortilla with oil, and flip to grill the other side.

YIELD: 2 servings

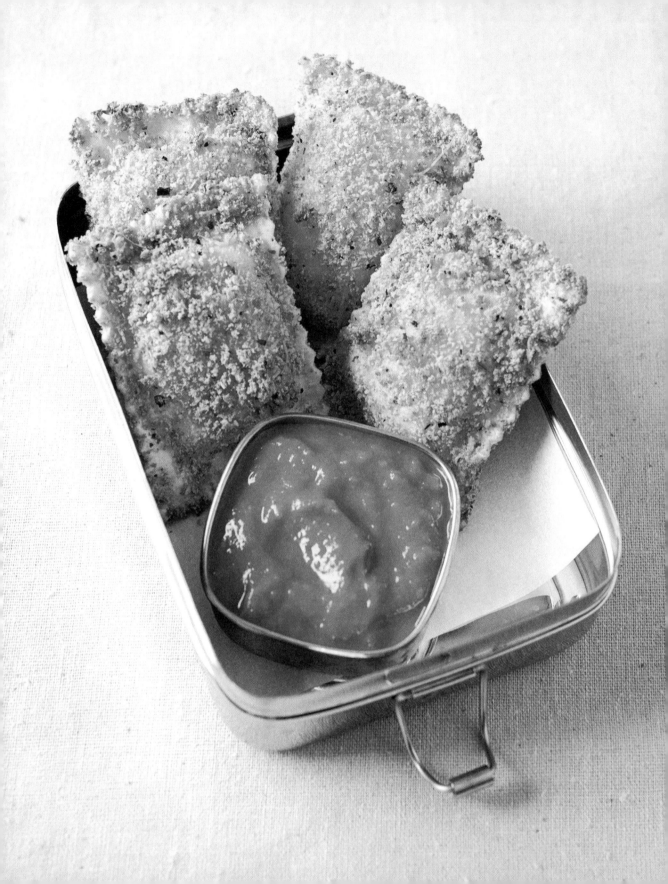

Baked Raviolis

There is a popular restaurant that serves fried raviolis as an appetizer. My daughter tried them once and loved them. Not wanting to eat fried foods at home (not to mention the mess of frying anything), I decided to bake them instead. This recipe was an all-around success!

1½ cups (175 g) plain Panko bread crumbs

¾ cup (90 g) plain bread crumbs

¼ teaspoon salt

2 teaspoons (4 g) Italian seasoning

1 tablespoon (5 g) grated Parmesan cheese

3 eggs, beaten

24 frozen cheese raviolis

Olive oil spray

Preheat the oven to 425°F (220°C), and line a large baking sheet with parchment paper.

In a shallow bowl, mix the bread crumbs, salt, Italian seasoning, and Parmesan cheese. In a large bowl, beat the eggs. Set aside.

In a medium saucepan, bring water to a boil, cook the raviolis for 3 minutes, drain and allow them to cool for 5 for 10 minutes.

Begin the breading process by adding 4 raviolis at a time to the beaten eggs, and flip to coat. Transfer to the Parmesan and breadcrumb mixture, and toss to coat well. Place on the baking sheet.

Repeat the breading process with the remaining ravioli. Coat lightly with the olive oil spray and bake for 15 minutes.

Serve with ¼ cup (60 g) Veggie Tomato Sauce (page 144).

For a school lunch: Make these ravioli for dinner the night before. Double this recipe if necessary. In the morning, lightly warm the ravioli and pack in a lunchbox. They are meant to be eaten at room temperature.

YIELD: 24 baked raviolis

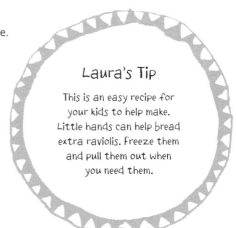

Laura's Tip

This is an easy recipe for your kids to help make. Little hands can help bread extra raviolis. Freeze them and pull them out when you need them.

Pesto Pasta

This pasta is the base for many delicious lunches. Add veggies, chicken, or sundried tomatoes for a complete meal.

1 box (16 ounces, or 454 g) elbow or rotini pasta

½ cup (130 g) Homemade Pesto (page 174)

2 teaspoons (10 ml) lemon juice

½ cup (115 g) Greek yogurt

Cook the pasta according to the package directions, drain and set aside.

In a large bowl, combine the pesto, lemon juice, and yogurt. Fold the pasta into the pesto until all the pasta is evenly coated. Serve warm or cold.

For a school lunch: Fill a preheated thermos with warm pasta, or pack inside a lunch container to be eaten cold.

YIELD: 8 servings

Garden Fresh Pasta

Is it a salad? Is it a pasta bowl? It's both! Colorful, fresh, nutritious, and the perfect way to use leftovers!

¾ cup (105 g) cooked pasta

2 teaspoons (30 g) Homemade Pesto (page 174)

¼ cup (56 g) chopped fresh baby spinach

¼ cup (38 g) cherry tomatoes, halved

½ carrot, grated

1 teaspoon grated Parmesan cheese

Mix all ingredients in a bowl until the pesto is thoroughly distributed.

YIELD: 1 serving

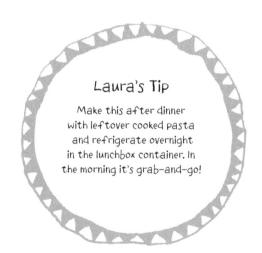

Laura's Tip

Make this after dinner with leftover cooked pasta and refrigerate overnight in the lunchbox container. In the morning it's grab-and-go!

Italian Pasta Salad

This easy-to-make pasta dish is one of my daughter's favorite lunches. It tastes just like pizza—a kid favorite for sure!

¾ cup (105 g) cooked pasta

4 or 5 slices pepperoni, chopped

2 ounces (40 g) mozzarella, cubed small

1½ tablespoons (15 g) black olives, sliced

¼ cup (45 g) cherry tomatoes, halved

2 teaspoons (30 ml) olive oil

Salt and pepper

In a bowl, combine all ingredients, adding salt and pepper to taste. Mix well until the oil evenly coats the salad.

YIELD: 1 serving

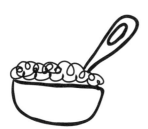

Greek Orzo Pasta Salad

This simple salad is filling, delicious, and full of Mediterranean flavor.

⅔ cup (75 g) whole wheat orzo pasta

1½ tablespoons (25 ml) olive oil

2 cups (60 g) baby spinach, chopped

½ cup (75 g) crumbled feta cheese

⅓ cup (48 g) raisins

¼ cup (25 g) finely chopped pitted black olives

2 tablespoons (30 ml) fresh lemon juice

Salt and pepper

Cook orzo according to package instructions, drain and empty into a bowl.

Toss the orzo with olive oil and mix it well to combine. Add the spinach, feta cheese, raisins, olives, lemon juice, and season with the salt and pepper to taste.

YIELD: 4 servings

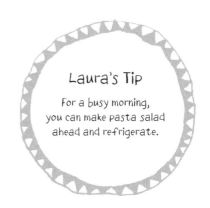

Laura's Tip

For a busy morning, you can make pasta salad ahead and refrigerate.

Neighborhood Meatballs

This is one of the first recipes my good friend Melissa shared with me when I moved into the neighborhood. It's a family favorite and a staple in both our homes.

For Meatballs:

4 ounces (120 g) Saltine crackers, finely crushed

1 pound (450 g) ground turkey or beef

½ pound (225 g) ground turkey sausage

¼ cup (6 g) parsley

3 eggs, beaten

2 teaspoons (6 g) garlic powder

½ teaspoon salt

1 teaspoon black pepper

¼ cup (25 g) grated Parmesan cheese

For Red Gravy:

3 tablespoons (45 ml) olive oil

1 small onion

2 cloves garlic, chopped

1 teaspoon salt

1 teaspoon black pepper

2 tablespoons (8 g) oregano

1 tablespoon (5 g) basil

3 cans (28 ounces, or 2.4 kg) crushed tomatoes

1 tablespoon (13 g) sugar

Preheat the oven to 400°F (200°C).

To make the meatballs: In a large bowl, combine the saltine crumbs, meat, parsley, eggs, garlic, salt, pepper, and Parmesan cheese. Mix with your hands until everything is evenly combined.

With your hands, form 24 meatballs. Place each meatball into a greased baking pan, cover with foil, and cook for 15 minutes. Flip them after 15 minutes, and remove the foil for the next 15 minutes.

To make the red gravy: While the meatballs are cooking, heat the olive oil over medium-high heat in an 8-quart (7.6 L) soup pot.

Add the onion and cook for 3 to 5 minutes, stirring occasionally, until translucent. Add the garlic, salt, pepper, oregano, and basil, and cook for a minute or two. Pour in the tomatoes and sugar. Stir, bring to a boil, and reduce the heat.

When the meatballs are done, carefully take them out and place them in the red gravy. Cook for an additional 30 to 45 minutes with the cover on to blend all the flavors.

YIELD: 8 servings

Laura's Tip

This recipe yields extra red gravy (or tomato sauce) and will be perfect for other dinners or lunches!

Meatball Dippers

Remember my awesome Neighborhood Meatballs your family loved for dinner? These fun dippers are hearty, filling, and one lunch option your kids will love.

6 to 8 small Neighborhood Meatballs (page 104)

3 or 4 thin slices (60 to 80 g) Parmesan Crostinis (page 169)

½ cup (123 g) tomato sauce from Neighborhood Meatballs

Skewer or place the meatballs in a lunch container. Pour and store warmed sauce in a leak-proof container or thermos. In a separate compartment or container, store crostinis.

YIELD: 1 serving

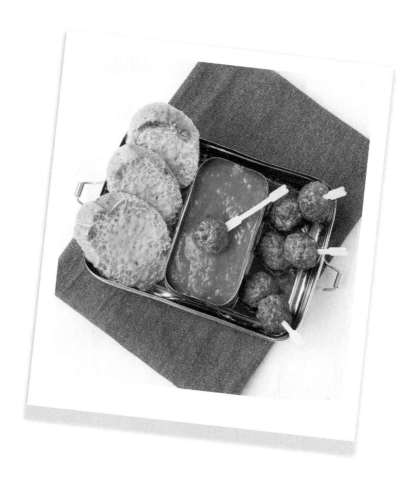

Olives and Feta Lego Pasta

One peek inside her thermos, and my daughter gets so excited when she finds this yummy pasta waiting for her. Good thing, because it's an easy dinner that yields leftovers!

1 pound (454 g) ditalini pasta

½ cup (120 ml) olive oil

1 lemon, juiced

1 can (6 ounces, or 170 g) whole black olives

One 4-ounce container (75 g) crumbled feta cheese

Kosher salt and freshly cracked black pepper

Bring a large pot of salted water to a boil over high heat. Add the pasta; reduce the heat, and cook until al dente, according to the package instructions, and drain.

While the pasta is cooking, in a medium bowl, whisk together the olive oil and lemon juice. Toss in the olives and feta.

Once the pasta is cooked, transfer it to the bowl. Toss all ingredients together until well combined. Add salt and pepper to taste, and serve.

For a school lunch: Warm the pasta leftovers and transfer to a preheated thermos.

YIELD: 6 servings

Arriba! Seasoning

Very similar to taco seasoning, but with a smoky flavor, less spice, and a whole lot of kid appeal.

3 tablespoons (23 g) chili powder

2 tablespoons (14 g) ground cumin

1 tablespoon (7 g) ground paprika

1½ teaspoons salt

2 teaspoons (4 g) black pepper

2 teaspoons (6 g) garlic powder

1 teaspoon onion powder

2 teaspoons (2 g) dried oregano

In a small bowl, combine all ingredients. Store in an airtight container.

YIELD: 9 tablespoons (69 g)

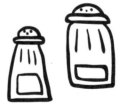

Arriba! Pasta Salad

Full of flavor and so easy to put together, this pasta dish is a family favorite!

For the Pasta Salad:

8 ounces (84 g) spiral pasta

2 cups (260 g) frozen corn

1 can (15 ounces, or 428 g) black beans, drained and rinsed

1 pint (180 g) grape or cherry tomatoes, halved,
or 1 can (411 g) fire-roasted tomatoes, drained

1 can (4 ounces, or 80 g) sliced black olives

½ cup (58 g) shredded Cheddar cheese

For the Dressing:

½ cup (115 g) Greek yogurt

2½ tablespoons (37 ml) lime juice

2 tablespoons (14 g) Arriba! Seasoning (page 106)

To make the pasta salad: Cook the pasta according to the package directions, drain and rinse. Set aside. In a large bowl, mix the corn, black beans, tomatoes, olives, and cheese.

Add the pasta to the bowl, and mix the ingredients well.

To make the dressing: In a large bowl, whisk all of the dressing ingredients until well combined.

Add the dressing to the pasta bowl. Using two large spoons, toss all ingredients together until everything is evenly coated with the dressing.

Serve immediately or refrigerate until ready to serve.

YIELD: 6 to 8 servings

Kitchen Note

I usually make this pasta early in the day so I have a quick dinner and use leftovers for lunch. Other days, however, I cook my pasta the night before, assemble the salad, and refrigerate for the next day. The longer the ingredients marinate, the better the flavor.

Southern Chicken Salad

This is one of the most visited recipes in my personal blog. It's a reader favorite and one of my family staples.

1 whole roasted chicken, meat off (about 2 cups [280 g])

3 tablespoons (45 ml) lemon juice

½ cup (115 g) mayonnaise

¼ teaspoon salt

½ teaspoon black pepper

1 teaspoon ground cumin

½ cup (60 g) finely chopped celery

Put the chicken in a food processor, and pulse a few times to roughly chop. Then continue pulsing for another 30 seconds until the chicken is finely chopped.

Note: If you turn on the food processor and let it go, your chicken will become a paste instead of finely chopped. So be sure to pulse the chicken for best results.

In a large bowl, combine the lemon juice, mayonnaise, salt, pepper, and cumin, and mix well until thoroughly combined.

Add the chicken to the bowl, and fold with a spatula. Fold in the celery.

YIELD: 6 servings

Dad's Tuna Pasta Salad

When I first met my husband, he ate tuna nearly every day for lunch. After a while, I couldn't take his daily tuna salad and crackers anymore, so I began to get creative by including anything we had in our fridge. This is now one of his favorite tuna salad combinations.

1½ cups (203 g) cooked pasta

⅓ cup (50 g) cherry tomatoes, sliced in half

¼ cup (25 g) ripe olives

¼ cup (33 g) frozen corn, thawed

1 tablespoon (15 ml) olive oil

5 ounces (142 g) tuna, can or pouch, drained

Salt and pepper

In a large bowl, combine all ingredients until the pasta is covered with the oil and the ingredients are evenly distributed. Season with the salt and pepper to taste. Pack in a lunch container.

YIELD: 2 servings

Mexican Pasta Salad

This is my go-to pasta salad after our usual Taco Tuesdays dinner. Full of flavor and easy to eat, it's perfect for a school lunch.

1 cup (140 g) cooked pasta of choice

1 ounce (20 g) Cheddar cheese

2 tablespoons (18 g) cooked ground beef or chicken, cut small

1 tablespoon (6 g) sliced ripe olives

2 tablespoons (33 g) mild salsa

1 tablespoon (6 g) corn

1 teaspoon olive oil

Dash each of salt and pepper

Mix all ingredients in a bowl. Toss well to evenly coat with the oil and seasonings.

YIELD: 1 serving

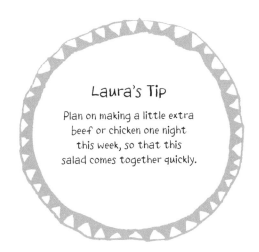

Laura's Tip

Plan on making a little extra beef or chicken one night this week, so that this salad comes together quickly.

Avocado Tuna Salad

When my kids start school, the temperature outside is still well into the '90s. Looking for a way to make tuna salad without mayonnaise led to using one of my favorite superfoods—avocados!

1 avocado

1 lemon, juiced

1 tablespoon (120 g) celery, finely chopped

Salt and pepper

1 can (6 ounces, or 170 g) water-packed tuna, drained

Cut the avocado in half. Remove the pit, and scoop out the avocado flesh into a bowl.

With a fork, coarsely mash the avocado. Add the lemon juice, celery, salt and pepper to taste, and mix well. Fold in the tuna, and combine.

For a school lunch: Pack the salad in a small container with a lid. Serve with baked corn chips and veggies. Alternatively, you can use the tuna salad to fill a wrap or a sandwich.

YIELD: 2 servings

No Mayo Egg Salad

I love substituting plain Greek yogurt in recipes where we would traditionally use mayonnaise. My kids don't mind the substitution, and I feel good about the extra probiotics, calcium, and protein.

4 hard-boiled eggs, diced

1 tablespoon (11 g) Dijon mustard

1 teaspoon (3 g) ground paprika

1 tablespoon (3 g) chives, chopped (optional)

3 tablespoons (45 g) Greek yogurt

Salt and pepper

In a bowl, combine all ingredients and mix thoroughly. Add salt and pepper to taste. Cover and refrigerate.

For a school lunch: Pack in a divided container with crackers or make it into a sandwich or wrap.

YIELD: 2 servings

Big Jim's Chicken Salad

This recipe comes from our friend Jim who shared his favorite version of chicken salad that he's enjoyed since he was a kid. It has since become one of our favorites as well.

1 tablespoon (15 ml) fresh lemon juice

¼ cup (60 g) mayonnaise

1 cup (140 g) finely diced cooked chicken

1 celery rib, finely diced

1 apple, peeled and diced small

2 slices bacon (15 g), cooked and crumbled

1 tablespoon (9 g) slivered almonds, chopped small (optional)

In a bowl, combine the lemon juice and mayonnaise. Toss in the chicken, celery, apple, bacon, and almonds. Mix well until all ingredients are evenly coated with the dressing.

For a school lunch: Serve this chicken salad with whole-grain crackers, or stuff it inside pita bread.

YIELD: 2 servings

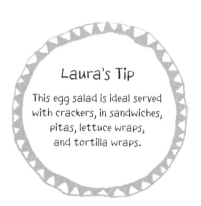

Laura's Tip

This egg salad is ideal served with crackers, in sandwiches, pitas, lettuce wraps, and tortilla wraps.

Veggie Meat Loaf

"Mom! There's green and orange stuff in here!" Oh, the confetti sprinkles you mean?

1 cup (130 g) carrots, finely chopped

½ zucchini (60 g), chopped

1 handful spinach, finely chopped

½ onion, chopped

2 cloves garlic, chopped

1 cup (115 g) bread crumbs

1 tablespoon (2 g) Italian seasoning

½ teaspoon black pepper

1½ pounds (340 g) ground turkey or beef

2 eggs

1 can (8 ounces, or 245 g) tomato sauce

3 tablespoons (48 g) barbecue sauce

Preheat the oven to 325°F (170 °C), and lightly grease a 9-inch (23 cm) loaf pan.

In a food processor or mini chopper, chop the carrots, zucchini, spinach, onion, and garlic until finely chopped. Place in a large bowl.

Add the bread crumbs, Italian seasoning, pepper, turkey, and eggs. Using your hands, combine the ingredients until they are all well mixed.

Pack the mixture into the loaf pan. Combine the tomato sauce and barbecue sauce, and pour over the meat mixture.

Bake for 1 hour to 1 hour 15 minutes. Oven times and temperatures will vary, so check for doneness after 50 minutes by using an instant-read thermometer. Turkey is cooked at 165°F (74°C), and beef at 160°F (71°C).

YIELD: 6 servings

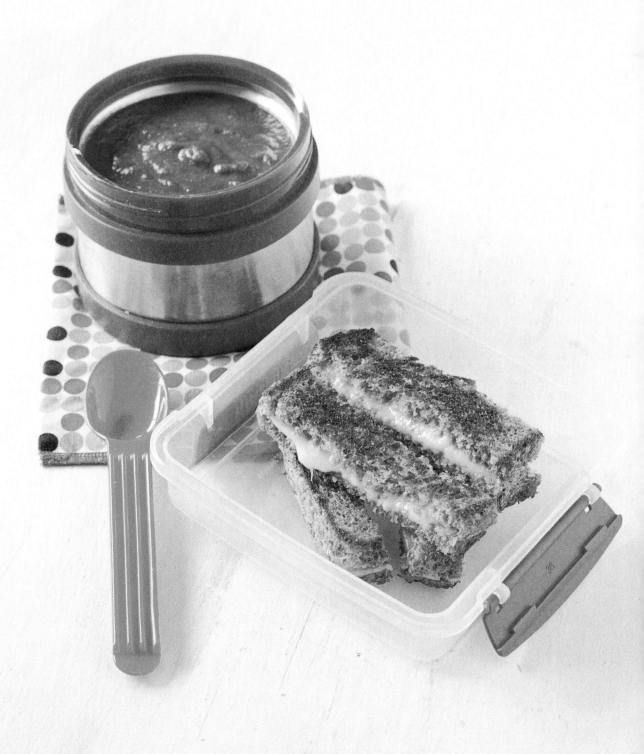

◄ Grilled Cheese Dippers

My daughter says "dipping is a lot more fun when cheese is involved." You know what? I must admit that I agree with her.

Butter, for grilling

2 slices whole-grain bread

2 slices (40 g) white Cheddar cheese

Butter one side of both bread slices; flip over onto a cutting board. Place the cheese on one slice of the bread and close the sandwich with the second slice.

Place the cheese sandwich, buttered side down, on a skillet over medium heat. Grill for 2 to 3 minutes, until the cheese has begun to melt, and the bread is golden brown. Press down with a spatula, flip, and grill the second side. Remove onto a cutting board.

Allow the sandwich to cool for 5 minutes, cut into narrow strips, and pack in a lunch container.

For a school lunch: Try serving it with Tomato Veggie Soup (page 150).

YIELD: 1 serving

Kitchen Note

Let the grilled sandwich cool down before slicing and packing it in the lunchbox. If you cut it too soon and pack it while it's still hot, the bread will be soggy by lunchtime.

Spaghetti Tacos

If your kids like "all things crunchy" like mine do, these spaghetti tacos are certain to be a lunchbox favorite. It's a crazy combo, but kids love it.

2 hard taco shells

1 cup (140 g) leftover spaghetti mixed with Veggie Tomato Sauce (page 144)

1 tablespoon (5 g) Parmesan cheese

Warm the taco shells in a toaster oven. Lightly warm the spaghetti.

Fill each taco shell with ½ cup (70 g) spaghetti. Sprinkle with the cheese.

For a school lunch: Pack spaghetti tacos in a big-enough lunch container so that they are able to lay flat. Otherwise, consider sending spaghetti separately, and have your child stuff the taco.

YIELD: 1 serving

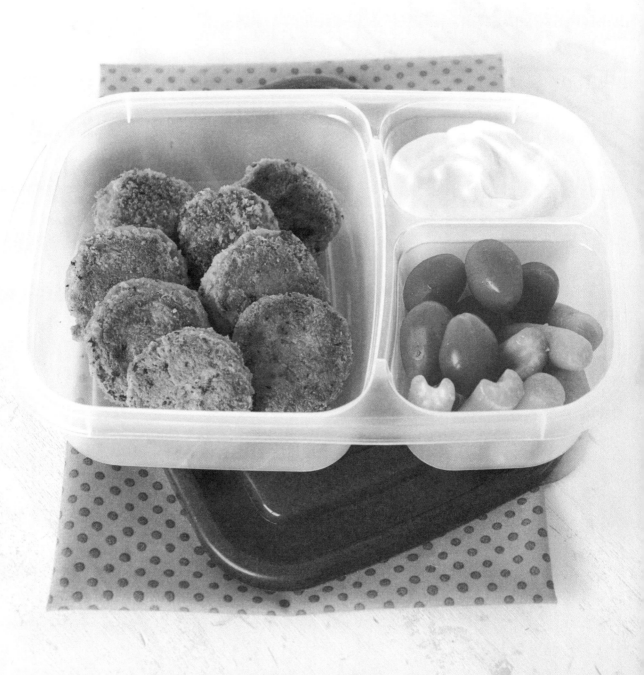

Lunchbox Falafels

I love the versatility of these falafels. Easy to make and great to eat at room temperature, they're perfect to have in the fridge (or uncooked in the freezer) for a convenient and healthy lunch.

½ cup (375 g) dry chickpeas, soaked overnight, or 1 cup (240 g) canned chickpeas

2 teaspoons (14 g) ground cumin

½ teaspoon ground coriander

1 or 2 cloves garlic, minced

1 parsley sprig, minced

1 small onion, chopped fine

1½ tablespoons (45 ml) freshly squeezed lemon juice

3 tablespoons (21 g) bread crumbs

Drain and rinse the chickpeas that were soaking overnight, or rinse the canned chickpeas.

In a food processor, pulse the chickpeas with all the ingredients until it becomes a smooth thick paste.

With wet hands, form the dough into small balls, the size of a large walnut. Press down to form 1½-inch (3.8 cm) patties. If the mixture is too sticky, add a little more bread crumbs. If it's too dry, add a tablespoon (15 ml) or two of water.

Cook the falafels in an oiled pan over medium-high heat for 3 to 4 minutes each side, or until brown. Remove onto a paper towel–lined plate.

Serve with Greek Yogurt Dip (page 177).

For a school lunch: In the morning, toast the falafels in a toaster oven, baking oven, or a pan. Pack inside a lunch container.

YIELD: 12 to 15 falafels

Olive Strips

These flavorful sandwich strips taste just like Mediterranean pizza—but without all the work!

1½ tablespoons (25 g) cream cheese

2 slices whole-grain bread

1 tablespoon (10 g) Olive Salad (page 174)

Spread the cream cheese on both slices of bread. Distribute the olive salad on one slice of the bread, and close the sandwich. Cut vertically into strips.

YIELD: 1 serving

Easy Peasy Frittata

I used to think frittatas were difficult to make because they sounded so fancy. This couldn't be further from the truth! They are easy to make and don't require flipping—which, for someone as messy as I am in the kitchen, is a good thing.

10 large eggs

⅓ cup (80 ml) milk

½ teaspoon salt

1 cup (130 g) frozen green peas

½ cup (58 g) shredded, sharp Cheddar cheese

2 tablespoons (28 g) butter

In a medium bowl, combine the eggs, milk, and salt. Whisk until well blended. Mix in the frozen peas and cheese.

In a 12-inch (30.5 cm) skillet, melt the butter over medium-low heat. Swirl the pan around to evenly distribute the butter over the entire bottom and sides of pan.

Pour the egg mixture into the pan and, using a rubber spatula, give the mixture a quick stir to distribute the peas evenly.

Turn the heat to low. Allow the egg mixture to cook without stirring, about 5 minutes. Meanwhile, preheat your oven's broiler. Once the edges are cooked, and the center and top are still semiliquid, transfer the skillet to the broiler and continue to cook until the top and center are fully cooked, about 4 minutes.

Remove from the oven, and allow the frittata to cool before slicing.

For a school lunch: Place one slice of frittata inside of a lunchbox.

YIELD: 6 servings

Laura's Tip

Remember to use an oven mitt when removing the pan from the oven. It will be quite hot! This lunch can be made ahead of time, stored in the refrigerator for up to three days, and enjoyed at room temperature.

CHAPTER 4

ADD SOME FUN: INTERACTIVE LUNCHES FOR PICKY EATERS

Kids love playing with their food, and healthy
food should be fun to eat!

This section helps you to find ways to sneak in more veggies,
to re-create some of those packaged lunches from the store
using healthy ingredients, and to introduce new foods in fun
and interactive ways. Kids also love to assemble their own
lunches, and this section will help to inspire both of you.

Remember that most of the time you'll need to
introduce a food in several different ways in order for
your child to learn to love it. Do your best and the
recipes in this book will take care of the rest.

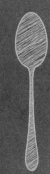

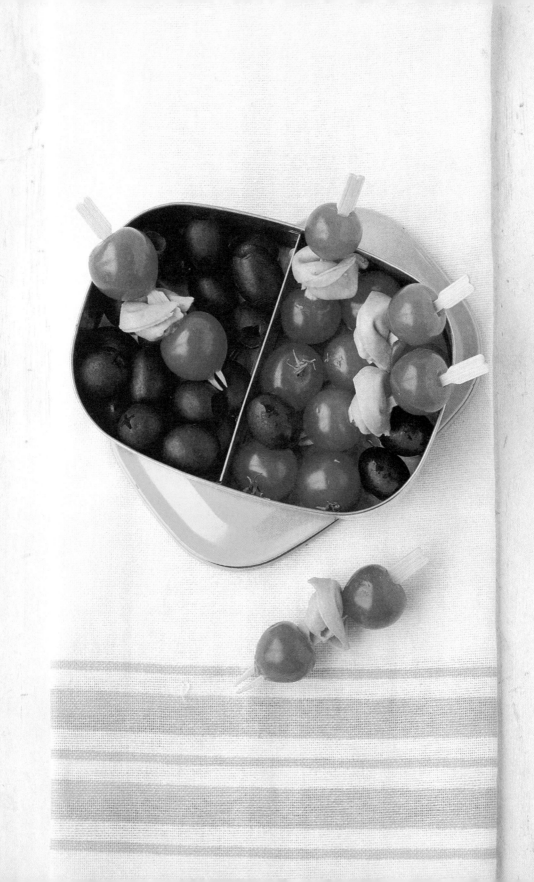

◀ Tortellini Swords

Last night's leftover tortellini becomes an easy-to-eat and delicious lunch.

½ cup (70 g) cooked tortellini

½ cup (75 g) cherry tomatoes

¼ cup (25 g) black olives

Using rounded-edge skewers or bento picks, alternate skewering tortellini, tomatoes, cheese, and olives.

Alternatively, if you don't have skewers, mix all ingredients in a bowl. Drizzle with olive oil, and make it into a salad.

YIELD: 1 serving

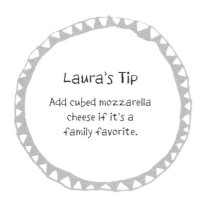

Laura's Tip

Add cubed mozzarella cheese if it's a family favorite.

Veggie Skewers

Stick veggies on a "sword," and you'll be surprised that this just might be the trick to get them to eat their veggies!

⅓ cup (50 g) cherry tomatoes

¼ cup (40 g) fresh mini mozzarella balls

⅓ avocado, pitted and cubed

½ tablespoon (8 g) Homemade Pesto (page 174)

¼ cup (56 g) Greek Hummus (page 175)

2 or 3 Parmesan Crostinis (page 169)

Using rounded-edge skewers or bento picks, alternate skewering tomatoes, mozzarella, and avocados. In two small lidded containers, pack the pesto and hummus.

Assemble all items in a compartmentalized lunch container, making sure the crostinis are in their own compartment.

YIELD: 1 serving

Real Chicken Nuggets

My friend, Cristi Messersmith, created a kid-friendly nugget recipe that her son, who has autism, would eat. It had to be a protein-rich version with a texture similar to the fast-food nuggets that was healthy, had real ingredients, and could be made in big batches. These are as close as it gets, and I'm thankful she shared her recipe with us.

1 teaspoon creole seasoning (or your favorite seasoning), divided

½ teaspoon garlic powder

¼ teaspoon black pepper

1 pound (450 g) ground chicken

¼ cup (20 g) old-fashioned oats

¼ cup (25 g) grated Parmesan cheese, divided

¾ cup (90 g) bread crumbs

Olive oil or cooking spray

Preheat the oven to 375°F (190°C).

In a small ramekin, mix creole seasoning, garlic powder, and pepper.

In large bowl, combine the chicken, oats, half the Parmesan, and half of the seasoning mixture. Knead well to combine.

With wet hands to prevent sticking, form a small ball of chicken mixture. Press into a cookie cutter for shaped nuggets or flatten with your fingers for a basic nugget shape.

In small bowl, combine the bread crumbs with the remaining seasoning mix and cheese. Press the nuggets into the bread crumb mixture and turn over, patting the crumbs into the surface to coat evenly. Arrange the nuggets on a parchment-lined baking sheet. Lightly spray the nuggets with cooking spray or olive oil for a crispier crust. Bake for 15 to 18 minutes, turning once, and checking for doneness by inserting an instant-read thermometer. The temperature should be 165°F (78°C).

For a school lunch: Warm nuggets in the toaster oven, pan, or broiler for a few minutes. Place in a lunchbox with a favorite dipping sauce. My daughter enjoys these at room temperature; but if keeping them warm is a concern, send them inside a thermos.

YIELD: 24 nuggets

Kitchen Note

When you shape them, don't make them too flat, or they will overcook. Thicker is better in this case. To freeze, flash-freeze nuggets, uncooked, on the baking sheet for one hour. Once frozen, transfer to a freezer ziplock bag to store.

Spaghetti Cupcakes

There's something magical about cupcakes—they make leftover spaghetti much more appealing.

8 ounces (227 g) uncooked spaghetti, or 4 to 5 cups (560 to 700 g) cooked leftover spaghetti

4 eggs, beaten

¼ teaspoon black pepper

1½ cups (368 g) Veggie Tomato Sauce (page 144)

2 cups (230 g) shredded mozzarella cheese

½ cup (50 g) grated Parmesan cheese + additional for sprinkling

Preheat the oven to 375°F (190°C) and grease a standard cupcake pan.

Cook the spaghetti according to package directions.

In a large bowl, whisk the eggs and pepper. Add tomato sauce, mozzarella, ½ cup (50 g) of the Parmesan, and spaghetti. Combine until everything is thoroughly coated.

Divide the spaghetti mixture evenly into cupcake pan wells. Bake for 12 to 15 minutes. Let stand 5 minutes before serving. Sprinkle with additional Parmesan.

For a school lunch: Lightly warm spaghetti cupcakes in the morning. These are meant to be eaten at room temperature, but if your child prefers them hot, insert them in a thermos. (I can usually fit 2 or 3 cupcakes stacked inside our thermos.)

YIELD: 4 servings

Build Your Own Pizza Lunch

I can see the kid appeal to making your own pizza. And by making your own pizza assembly lunchbox, you'll make sure the ingredients are fresh, more nutritious, and have a lot more toppings!

1 English muffin, split

2 ounces (55 g) Veggie Tomato Sauce (page 144) or pizza sauce

¼ cup (30 g) shredded mozzarella or mild Cheddar cheese

Toppings of choice: pepperoni, ham, black olives

Lightly toast the muffin.

Store the tomato sauce in a small leak-proof container and the cheese in a separate container. Include the toppings in other small containers.

YIELD: 1 serving

Kitchen Note

If you don't have small containers with lids, a compartmentalized lunchbox works very well. With younger kids, you might want to assemble the pizzas ahead of time and toast them in the toaster oven or broiler for 2 minutes.

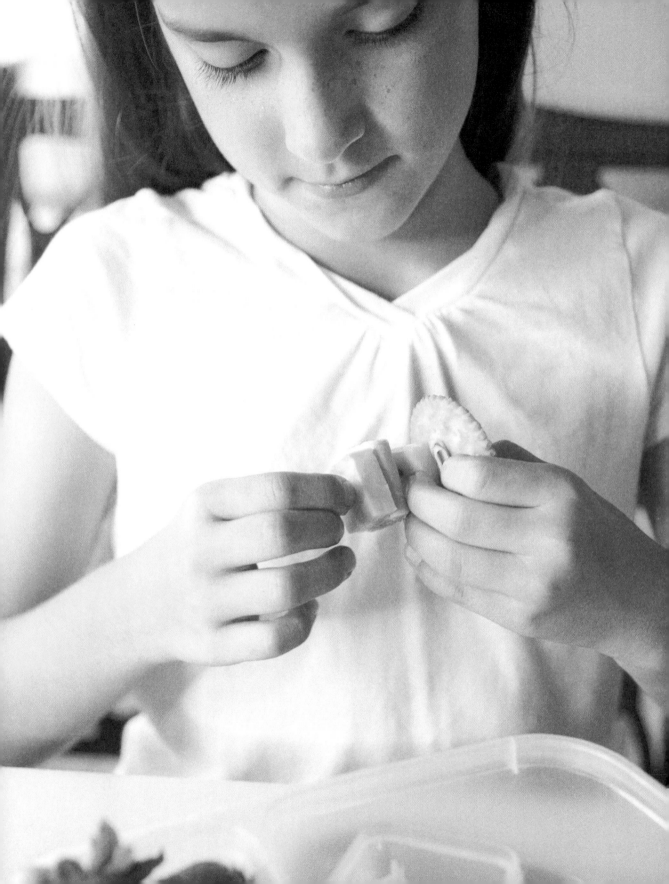

Ham and Cheese Swords

My daughter loves swords. The ingredient possibilities are endless but oftentimes, she requests the most basic, yet her favorite, combination.

3 slices (60 g) honey ham

2 ounces (40 g) Cheddar cheese, cubed

6 to 8 whole-grain crackers

On a cutting board, roll the ham tightly. Slice it into ½-inch (1.3 cm) pieces.

Alternate skewering the ham and cheese through toothpicks or bento picks.

For a school lunch: Serve the swords with whole-grain crackers, fresh fruit, and veggies.

YIELD: 1 serving

Kitchen Note

This is a great lunch to pack ahead of time. Make sure you store whole-grain crackers in a separate compartment or container so that they do not absorb moisture from the other food items.

Build Your Own Roman Army Boats

For the kid who won't eat chicken Caesar salad, because Roman Army Boats are a lot more fun.

⅓ cup (47 g) oven-roasted chicken, chopped

1 hard-boiled egg, chopped

1 tablespoon (15 ml) Caesar dressing

1 tablespoon (5 g) grated Parmesan cheese

4 to 6 hearts of romaine leaves

In a small bowl, combine the chicken, egg, and dressing. Sprinkle with the cheese. Serve on the lettuce leaves.

For a school lunch: There are two ways to pack this lunch. Make the salad, pack it in a small container with a lid, and pack the lettuce leaves separately. The second option is to preassemble the lettuce cups in a rectangular lunchbox.

YIELD: 1 serving

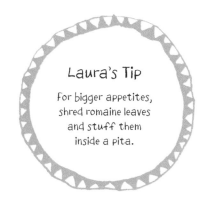

Laura's Tip

For bigger appetites, shred romaine leaves and stuff them inside a pita.

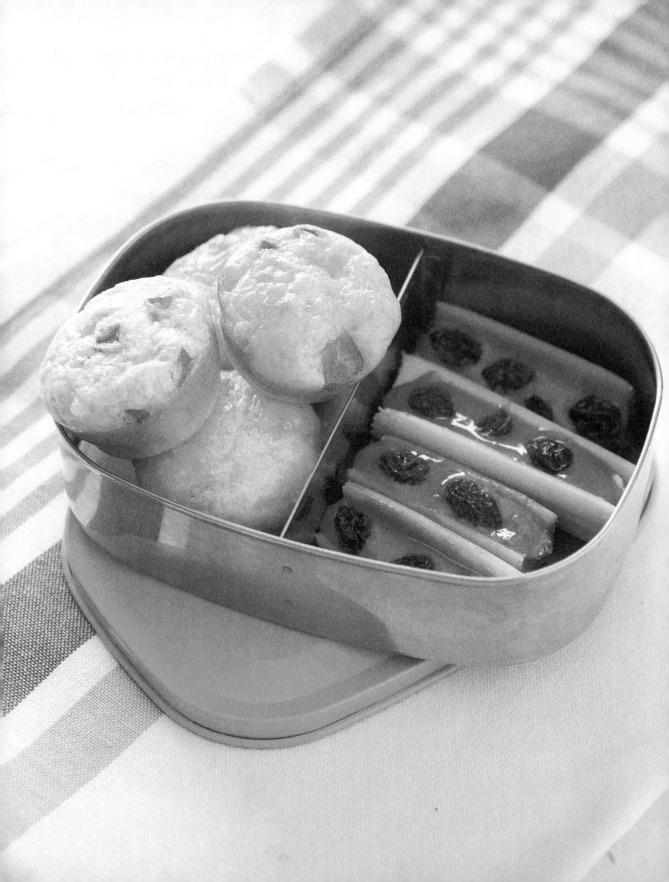

◄ Mini Quiches

Easy, portable, perfectly portioned—all the things kids love in a tiny bite. Mix up the "add ins," and this recipe yields hundreds of options.

6 eggs

¼ cup (60 g) plain Greek yogurt

3 tablespoons (45 ml) milk

½ cup (75 g) ham, diced

1 cup (120 g) shredded Cheddar cheese

¼ teaspoon salt

¼ teaspoon black pepper

Preheat the oven to 350°F (180°C) and grease a mini muffin pan.

In a large bowl, whisk the eggs, yogurt, and milk. Add the ham, cheese, salt, and pepper.

Distribute the mixture evenly into the pan. Bake for 15 to 18 minutes. Allow the quiches to cool in the pan before carefully removing with a small knife or spatula.

For a school lunch: In the morning, reheat the quiches or pack cold. They will be room temperature by lunch.

YIELD: 24 mini quiches

Build Your Own Parfait

Your kids will be the envy of the lunch table with this lunch!

1 cup (230 g) low-fat vanilla yogurt

½ cup (75 g) mixed berries (sliced strawberries and blueberries)

1 tablespoon (5 g) Lunchbox Granola (page 44)

1 Whole Wheat Waffle (page 44)

Pour the yogurt inside a chilled thermos. Top with the berries, and sprinkle with the granola. Close the thermos.

For a school lunch: Serve the parfait with a waffle with a side of maple syrup, Easy Freezer Jam (page 170), or White Chocolate Peanut Butter (page 173).

YIELD: 1 serving

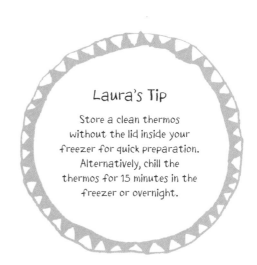

Laura's Tip

Store a clean thermos without the lid inside your freezer for quick preparation. Alternatively, chill the thermos for 15 minutes in the freezer or overnight.

Mac and Cheese Bites

Mac and cheese is an all-time kid favorite! And this simple recipe makes it easy to pack for lunch.

6 ounces (70 g) uncooked small pasta shells

1 egg

1 tablespoon (15 ml) milk

¾ cup (86 g) shredded Cheddar cheese

Preheat the oven to 350°F (180°C) and grease a mini muffin pan.

Cook the pasta according to the package directions. Allow it to cool to room temperature.

In a large bowl, beat the egg. Add the milk and cheese, mix, and add the pasta. Toss to combine.

Distribute the pasta mixture evenly in the wells of the pan. Bake for 15 to 20 minutes, until golden brown. Remove from the oven, allow them to cool for 5 minutes, remove from the pan, and serve.

For a school lunch: In the morning, warm the bites and either pack them in a preheated thermos or in a lunch container.

YIELD: 24 bite-size pieces

Kitchen Note

For extra nutrition, add up to ½ cup (75 g) chopped veggies to the mix, such as broccoli or peas.

Monkey Towers

Who wants a boring PB&J when you can build a tower of nut butter fun! This is a great lunch to have your kids help you put together. In fact, my son loves to make these cracker bites into stackable towers at lunch. Of course, I always remind him that his job is to take the tower down—right down into his tummy, that is!

2 tablespoons (520 g) peanut butter

10 whole wheat round crackers

½ banana, sliced

Spread a thin layer of peanut butter on all crackers. Top with 1 slice of banana, and top with another cracker, pressing gently.

YIELD: 1 serving

Veggie Nuggets

Designed for nugget-lovers and picky eaters everywhere, these delicious meat-free veggie bites are a real kid (and mom) pleaser.

½ large cauliflower

1 broccoli crown

3 eggs

¾ cup (87 g) bread crumbs

½ cup (50 g) grated Parmesan cheese

2 teaspoons (12 g) Arriba! Seasoning

Salt and pepper

Steam the cauliflower and broccoli until they are cooked and soft. Rinse in cold water to stop the cooking process.

Preheat the oven to 375°F (190°C).

Place the cauliflower and broccoli inside a food processor. Pulse a few times, then turn on for a minute or two, until it's thoroughly combined.

Add the eggs, bread crumbs, cheese, seasoning, and add salt and pepper to taste to the veggie mixture. Give the food processor a few pulses until all the ingredients are evenly combined. If the veggie paste is too sticky, add additional bread crumbs. This will vary based on the size of your broccoli and cauliflower heads.

Using a cookie scoop or your hands to make small golf-ball-size nuggets, place the scoops onto a parchment-lined baking sheet. Bake for about 15 minutes until golden brown.

For a school lunch: Serve warmed veggie nuggets in a thermos or at room temperature in any lunchbox along with ¼ cup (61 g) of Veggie Tomato Sauce (page 144) in a small container with a lid for dipping.

YIELD: 36 to 48 nuggets

Kitchen Note

You can freeze uncooked nuggets on a baking sheet. Once frozen, transfer to a freezer bag. To bake, preheat the oven, and add 2 to 3 minutes to the baking time.

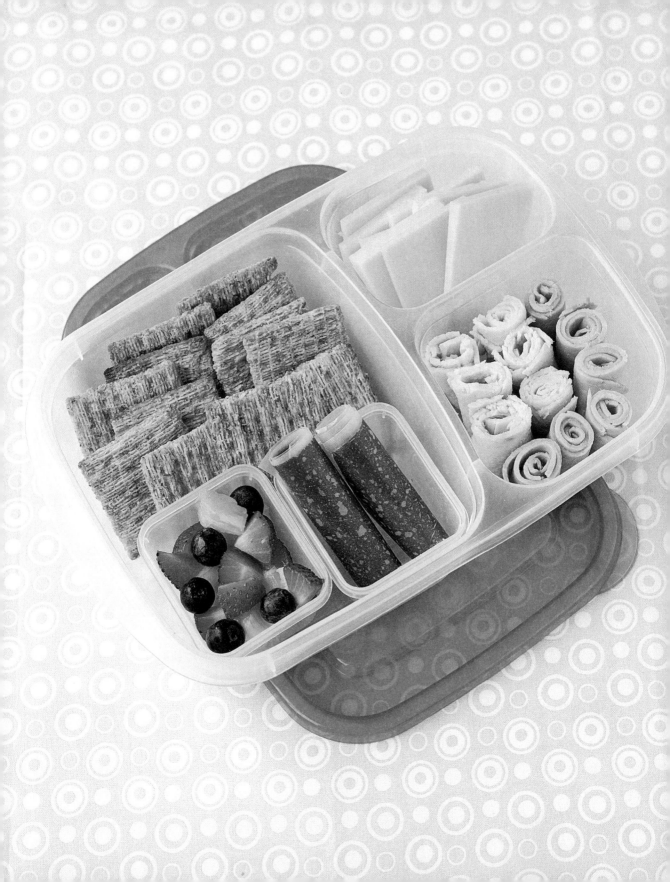

◀ The Original MOMable

This is the school lunch that started my own lunch revolution and built an entire community of parents who want fresh lunches for their kids. Easy to make, a kid favorite, and mine uses real ingredients.

2 ounces (40 g) white Cheddar cheese

2 slices (40 g) ham or turkey

8 whole-grain crackers

Strawberry Fruit Leather (page 84)

On a cutting board, cut the cheese into thin square pieces. Cut the ham in half, and fold into quartered pieces.

For a school lunch: Assemble all the ingredients in a lunchbox, making sure the crackers are in their own compartment so that they do not absorb moisture and get soggy. Add fresh fruit or veggies.

YIELD: 1 serving

Old School Cracker Stackers

Sometimes, kids find lunchbox joy in the simplest of things. For my son, it's licking the peanut butter and jelly after he twists these crackers open.

2 tablespoons (32 g) peanut butter

1 tablespoon (20 g) Easy Freezer Jam (page 170)

12 whole wheat round crackers

Spread peanut butter and jam on half of the crackers, close into a cracker sandwich.

YIELD: 1 serving

Laura's Tip

This is the perfect lunch for a rushed morning of when you have nothing left to pack, or you've run out of bread and everything else. Serve along with yogurt, fruit, and veggies for a complete lunch.

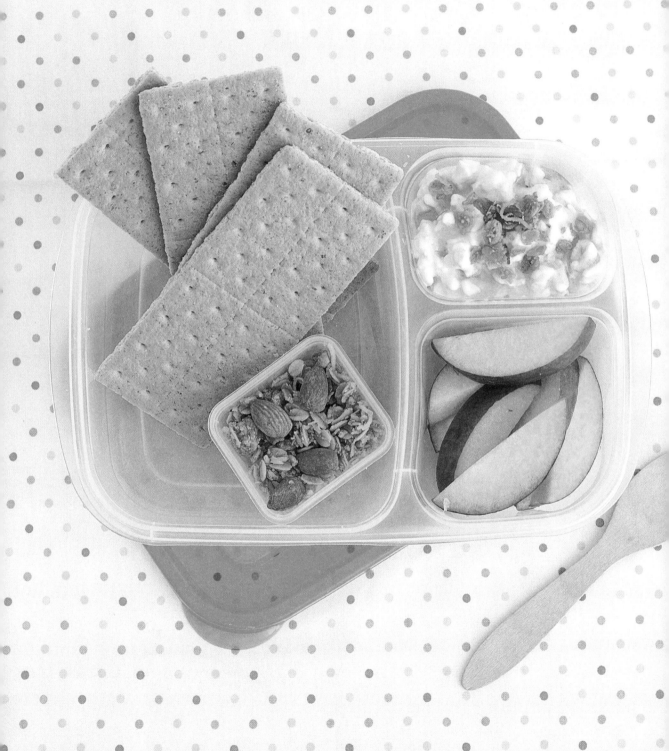

◀ Peach Cobbler Box

This lunchbox reminds me of summer, all year long.

½ cup (125 g) ricotta cheese

1 teaspoon honey

1 fresh peach, sliced

2 tablespoons (15 g) granola

4 graham crackers

Drizzle the ricotta with honey and top with the peaches.

Pack in a leak-proof container, or two separate leak-proof containers.

Store the granola and graham crackers separately, so that the dry ingredients do not get soggy by absorbing moisture from the wet ingredients.

YIELD: 1 serving

Monkey Hot Dog

It looks like a hot dog, but it's not! Fun, meat-free, and quick to assemble—these are just a few of the reasons this lunch is a winner!

1 whole-grain hot dog bun

2 tablespoons (32 g) peanut butter

1 banana

1 tablespoon (20 g) Easy Freezer Jam (page 170)

Spread the bun with the peanut butter and top with the banana. Spread the jam over the banana.

YIELD: 1 hot dog

Kitchen Note

Spread peanut butter and jelly on a hot dog bun, and pack an unpeeled banana in the lunchbox. Let your child assemble the hot dog at lunch.

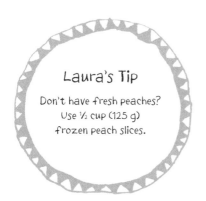

Laura's Tip

Don't have fresh peaches?
Use ½ cup (125 g)
frozen peach slices.

Quinoa Bites

These meat-free high-protein bites are perfect for nugget-loving kids.

½ cup (86 g) quinoa

1 cup (235 ml) broth or stock

2 cups (180 g) oat flour

½ cup (28 g) finely chopped fresh spinach

1 cup (110 g) finely grated carrots

½ cup (50 g) grated Parmesan cheese

1 egg

¼ cup (60 ml) olive oil

⅓ cup (80 ml) milk

1½ teaspoons baking powder

Cook the quinoa in the broth according to the package directions. Allow it to cool.

In a large bowl, combine the oat flour and quinoa. Add the spinach and carrots, and toss to combine.

In a medium-size bowl, mix the cheese, egg, olive oil, milk, and baking powder. Pour into the quinoa–veggie mixture. Mix until a thick batter is formed.

Preheat the oven to 350°F (180°C). Line a standard-size cupcake pan with paper liners (or grease the sides well) and fill each about halfway full with batter. Bake for 20 to 25 minutes, until golden brown. Remove from the oven, and allow the bites to cool slightly before serving.

YIELD: 10 bites

Pesto Lover's Box ▶

When my youngest (at seventeen months of age) began dipping everything in my homemade pesto, I began creating pesto "boxes" for lunch. So simple, fresh, and delicious!

¼ cup (65 g) Homemade Pesto (page 174)

¼ cup (57 g) whole ripe olives

½ cup (75 g) cherry tomatoes

2 ounces (30 g) mozzarella cheese, cubed

2 or 3 Parmesan Crostinis (page 169)

Assemble all the ingredients in a large lunchbox container, making sure that the pesto sauce is stored in a separate small leak-proof container.

YIELD: 1 serving

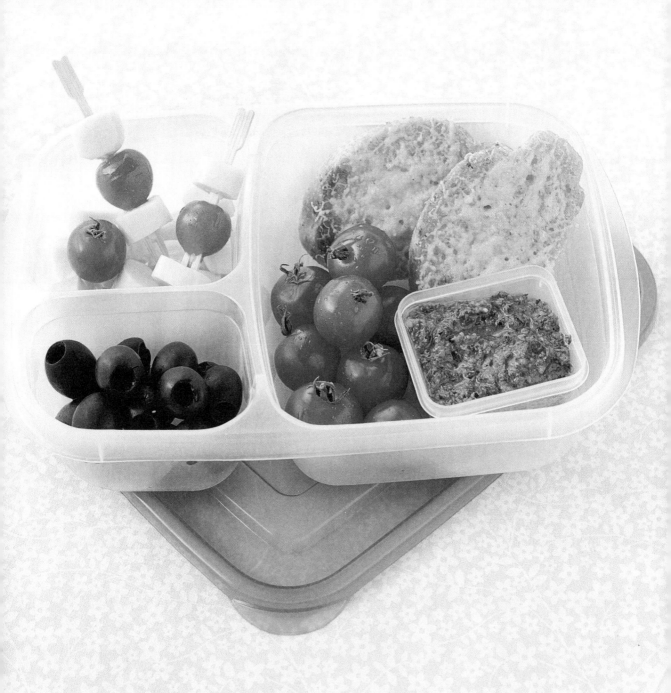

Baked Mozzarella Sticks

My kids love baked mozzarella sticks for dinner. Once, I packed the leftovers in the lunchbox, and they loved it! Straight out of the fridge, and into the lunchbox with my Veggie Tomato Sauce on the side.

12 sticks part-skim mozzarella string cheese

¼ cup (30 g) plain bread crumbs

¼ cup (12.5 g) Panko bread crumbs

2 teaspoons (3 g) grated Parmesan cheese

1½ tablespoons (3 g) Italian seasoning

¼ cup (32 g) all-purpose flour

1 large egg, beaten

Veggie Tomato Sauce (page 144)

Remove the wrappers and cut the cheese in half to get 24 pieces. Freeze the cheese until hard and frozen, about an hour. (This will allow you to bake them without melting.)

In a small shallow bowl, mix the bread crumbs, cheese, and Italian seasoning. In two other shallow bowls, place all-purpose flour and egg. Line up your bowls assemblyline style.

Line a baking sheet with parchment paper, and grease a cookie cooling rack. Place the greased rack on top of the lined baking sheet.

Remove the frozen cheese sticks, and immediately dip the sticks in the flour, shaking off the excess, then into the egg, and then a coating of bread crumb mix, placing them on the greased rack.

Once all cheese sticks are breaded, freeze the rack for about 15 minutes or until you're ready to bake them. Of course, you can double this recipe and leave extras, uncooked, for future meals.

Preheat the oven to 400°F (200°C) and move the oven rack to the bottom shelf of your oven. Bake for 4 to 5 minutes, turn cheese sticks over, and bake an additional 4 to 5 minutes.

Remove from the oven, and serve with the tomato sauce.

YIELD: 24 mini cheese sticks

Kitchen Note

I like to purchase a few packages of mozzarella cheese sticks and bread them all at once, freeze and thaw out as I need them for dinner, or quickly bake in the morning for school lunches.

Baked Zucchini Fries

A local restaurant serves zucchini fries as part of their kid's menu. Wanting to replicate the one way my son will eat zucchini led to baking them at home. Alex's "green fries" are a hit at dinner and inside the lunchbox too.

¼ cup (31 g) all-purpose flour

1 teaspoon Arriba! Seasoning (page 106)

1 large egg, beaten

1 tablespoon (15 ml) milk

1 cup (115 g) Panko or regular bread crumbs

1 tablespoon (5 g) grated Parmesan cheese

3 small zucchini, sliced into fry shapes

Preheat the oven to 400°F (200°C). Line a baking sheet with parchment paper and grease a cookie cooling rack. Place the greased rack on the top of the lined baking sheet.

In a small bowl, mix the all-purpose flour and Arriba! Seasoning. In another bowl, mix the egg and the milk. In a third bowl, mix the bread crumbs and Parmesan cheese. Line up your bowls assembly line style.

First, dip each zucchini stick in the flour mix, followed by the egg mix, and the bread crumb mix last. Place on the rack. Bake for 20 to 24 minutes, until light brown and crispy.

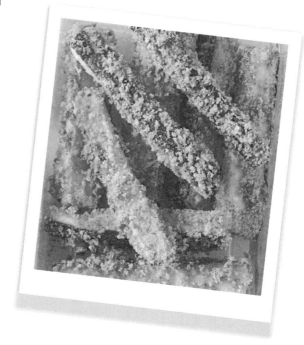

For a school lunch: I like to prepare these fries for dinner and use leftovers in our lunchboxes. In the morning, I warm them up in my toaster oven at 350°F (180°C) for 5 minutes. These are meant to be eaten at room temperature. Pack along with some Veggie Tomato Sauce (page 144) in a small leak-proof container.

YIELD: 30 to 40 fries

CHAPTER 5

FILL THE THERMOS: PORTABLE HOT LUNCHES

A thermos container will allow you to reuse leftovers and send hot foods to school.

Start by preheating the thermos. To preheat, bring water to a boil (either on the stovetop on in the microwave), fill the thermos container with the hot water, and let it sit for about five minutes. Then, pour out the hot water and fill it with heated leftovers.

Remember that you are warming up the leftovers to be eaten 3 to 5 hours later. The contents will need to be heated to a boil, on the stove, or piping hot in the microwave prior to placing them inside the thermos.

In this section, I share some of my family's favorite recipes. Most of which yield leftovers your kids will love packed for lunch.

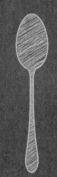

Tuna Quinoa Casserole

Creamy, cheesy, and full of flavor, this is one of the few ways my kids have tolerated quinoa.

1 cup (173 g) quinoa, dry

2 cups (470 g) vegetable stock

2 tablespoons (28 g) butter

2 tablespoons (16 g) flour

1 cup (120 ml) half and half or whole milk

1 cup (120 g) shredded, sharp Cheddar cheese

1 cup (115 g) mozzarella cheese, shredded

½ cup (40 g) Parmesan cheese, shredded

¼ teaspoon salt

¼ teaspoon black pepper

½ teaspoon ground cumin

1 cup (156 g) broccoli florets, thawed and finely chopped

½ cup (65 g) frozen corn

1 can (6 ounces, or 170 g) water-packed tuna, drained

Preheat the oven to 350°F (180°C).

Cook the quinoa in the vegetable stock by bringing it to a boil, reducing the heat, and simmering for 15 minutes, or until all liquid has been absorbed.

While the quinoa is cooking, melt the butter over medium heat in a large skillet. Add the flour, and whisk continuously for a couple of minutes until the mixture thickens. Slowly pour in the half and half, and whisk to combine while removing any lumps.

In a small bowl, combine the cheeses. Reserve half of the cheese, and add the rest to the pan slowly while stirring. Once the cheese is melted, add the salt, pepper, and cumin.

When the quinoa is done, add the quinoa to the cheese sauce. Stir in the broccoli, corn, and tuna.

Pour the quinoa into a casserole dish. Top with the reserved cheese, and bake for 12 minutes or until the cheese is melted and bubbly.

For a school lunch: Fill a preheated thermos with warmed casserole.

YIELD: 6 servings

Laura's Tip

Add 1 to 2 tablespoons (15 to 30 ml) of milk when heating up leftovers. It helps revive the sauce.

Dad's Fried Rice

My friend Jim is not only a father of two but also a fried rice connoisseur. He says there are no measurements to follow when making fried rice, just some simple rules, such as use leftover rice, don't skip the egg, add lots of "stuff" and be sure to make fried rice in a particular order. This recipe is easy and enables you to add a lot of delicious add-ins—a great way to utilize leftover veggies!

1 tablespoon (15 ml) vegetable oil

1 large egg, beaten

2 strips bacon, chopped

½ cup (70 g) cooked chicken, diced

1 cup (130 g) Asian stir-fry vegetables or 1 cup (130 g) peas, carrots, and baby corn mix, thawed

1 to 2 teaspoons (5 to 10 ml) soy or fish sauce

2 cups (330 g) cooked rice

In a large skillet, heat the oil over medium-high heat. Add the egg. Let it sit until it begins to bubble and an omelet forms. Flip over, and cook until done. Then, transfer to a small bowl.

Add the bacon to the skillet. Cook for 5 to 7 minutes, stirring occasionally. When the bacon pieces are cooked, add the chicken. Then add the vegetables and soy sauce, and cook for a couple of minutes until everything is warmed through.

Finally, add the rice and egg. Thoroughly mix everything together. Once the rice and egg are evenly distributed and seared, turn off the heat and serve.

YIELD: 3 servings

Bombay Rice ▶

My aunt made this rice for me, and I immediately loved the sweet and tangy flavors. So I asked her to write the recipe down for me to share. It's both delicious hot in a thermos, or served room temperature in a lunchbox.

1½ cups (360 ml) water

½ cup (120 ml) orange juice

1 cup (195 g) rice

¼ cup (60 g) pineapple chunks

⅓ cup (27 g) unsweetened, shredded coconut

⅓ cup (40 g) nuts, chopped, or ⅓ cup (48 g) raisins (optional)

Bring the water and juice to a boil, then add the rice and raisins. Lower the heat, cover, and simmer until all the liquid is absorbed, about 20 minutes.

With a fork, fluff the rice and fold in the pineapple chunks and coconut. Mix in the nuts or raisins, if using.

YIELD: 4 servings

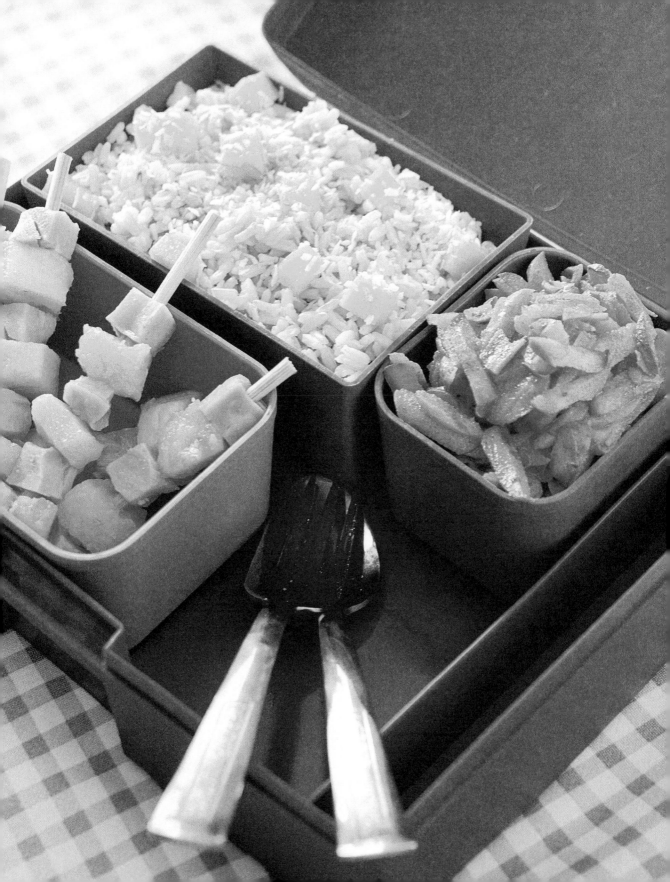

Stoplight Rice

My friend, Michelle Castañeda, has a knack for making fun food the pickiest of, eaters will love. This Stoplight Rice is a favorite among thousands in the MOMables community, and it's an easy recipe for sneaking in some veggies.

2 tablespoons (30 ml) vegetable oil

1 cup (185 g) long-grain white rice

1 clove garlic, minced

1 medium zucchini, grated

¼ red bell pepper, diced

1 small carrot, grated

Pinch of salt

2 cups (470 ml) low-sodium chicken broth

1 cup (115 g) shredded, sharp Cheddar cheese

Heat the oil in a medium saucepan over medium-high heat. Add the rice and garlic, and toss until all of the rice is coated with oil.

Add the zucchini, bell pepper, carrot, salt, and broth to the pot. Give everything a quick stir, and bring to a boil. Reduce the heat to simmer, and cook for 17 to 20 minutes until most of liquid has been absorbed.

Remove the pot from the heat completely, and stir in the cheese. Using a rubber spatula, fold the rice and cheese until it has melted and is thoroughly combined.

For a school lunch: Pack warm Stoplight Rice inside a preheated thermos.

YIELD: 4 servings

Bacon, Corn, and Avocado Macaroni

A great way to save money is to buy avocados in bulk. But when you do, that means finding creative ways to use them before they spoil. This amazing pasta dish is the delicious result of finding new ways to enjoy ripe, nutritious avocados.

2 ripe avocados, pitted and finely chopped

½ cup (65 g) frozen corn, thawed

4 slices bacon, cooked and chopped

1 lemon, juiced

½ teaspoon kosher salt

⅓ cup (34 g) grated Parmesan cheese

¼ teaspoon black pepper

2 tablespoons (30 ml) extra-virgin olive oil

8 ounces (105 g) elbow macaroni, uncooked

In a large bowl, mix the avocados, corn, bacon, lemon juice, salt, cheese, pepper, and oil. Cook the pasta according to the package directions, rinse and drain, and add it to the bowl.

Carefully fold the pasta, making sure all the ingredients are evenly distributed. Serve immediately.

For a school lunch: Fill a warmed thermos with the pasta.

YIELD: 4 servings

Creamy Avocado Pasta

My son loves this dish and calls it "superhero pasta." He claims it makes his tummy "big and full just like the Hulk's."

3 large, ripe avocados, pitted and flesh scooped from the skin

2 cloves garlic, minced, divided

3 tablespoons (45 ml) lemon juice

1 teaspoon lemon peel

Salt and pepper, to taste

1 tablespoon (15 ml) olive oil

1½ cups (270 g) cherry tomatoes, halved

12 ounces (75 g) mini penne pasta, cooked

½ cup (50 g) grated Parmesan cheese + additional for topping

Place the avocados in a food processor along with the half of the garlic, the lemon juice, and peel. Season with the salt and pepper, and blend until smooth.

In a large saucepan, place the olive oil and the remaining garlic. Cook the garlic over medium heat, until it turns golden. Add the tomatoes, and cook for about 5 minutes.

Add cooked pasta to the large saucepan. Give it a good stir to combine. Add the avocado mixture and cheese, toss well, and cook for another 2 minutes until the avocado sauce is creamy and warm.

Top with additional Parmesan cheese when serving.

For a school lunch: Fill a warmed thermos with the pasta.

YIELD: 6 servings

Peasy Tortellini

Leftover tortellini is my one of daughter's favorite lunches. The addition of some cheesy Alfredo sauce helps to hide her not-so-favorite vegetables.

1 cup (140 g) cooked tortellini

2 tablespoons (14 g) Homemade Alfredo Sauce (page 143)

2 tablespoons (16 g) frozen green peas

Mix all the ingredients in a bowl. Toss well to evenly coat with the sauce. Warm and pack in a thermos container.

YIELD: 1 serving

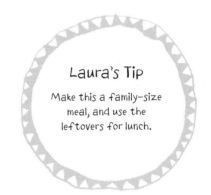

Laura's Tip

Make this a family-size meal, and use the leftovers for lunch.

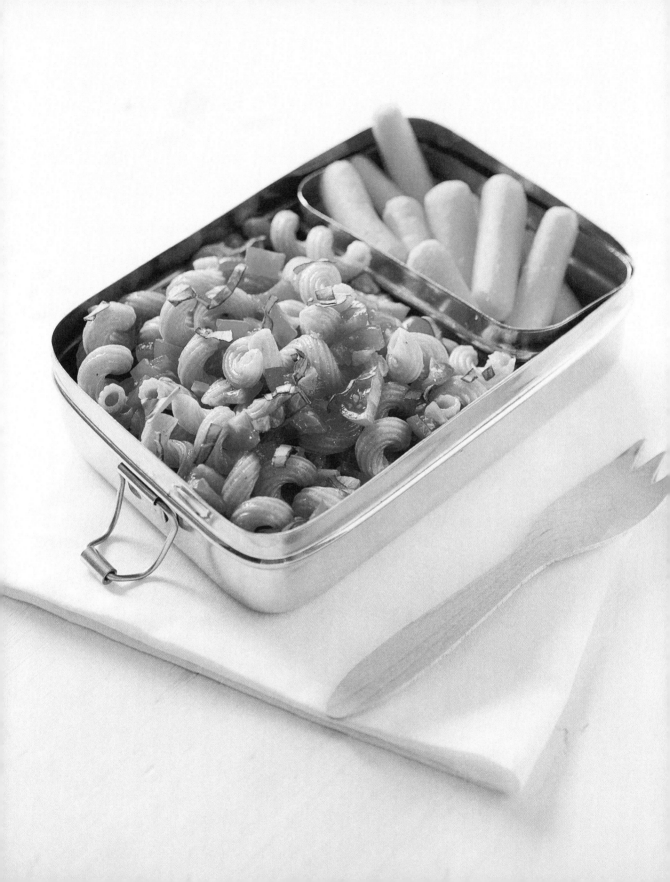

Margarita Pasta Salad

This salad is simple and delicious. Just like a Margarita pizza but with pasta!

¾ cup (102 g) cooked pasta

1 tablespoon (2.5 g) minced basil

¼ cup (45 g) cherry tomatoes, halved

2 teaspoons (30 ml) olive oil

Salt and pepper

In a large bowl, combine all the ingredients. Mix well until the oil evenly coats the pasta. Season with the salt and pepper to taste.

YIELD: 1 serving

Homemade Alfredo Sauce

Who knew that making your own Alfredo sauce was this easy! Ditch the jarred stuff and save money and increase nutrition with this homemade version. In fact, you probably already have all the ingredients on hand!

½ cup (112 g) butter

2 cups (475 ml) half and half or whole milk

2 teaspoons (6 g) garlic powder

2 tablespoons (15 g) cream cheese

½ cup (50 g) grated Parmesan cheese

Bring the butter, half and half, garlic, and cream cheese to a boil while stirring often. Turn down the heat, simmer, and stir for about 2 minutes.

Add the Parmesan, and stir until melted. Simmer the sauce (on your smallest burner) for 15 to 20 minutes until it thickens while stirring occasionally.

YIELD: About 2¾ cups (534 g)

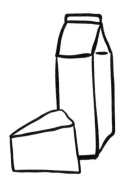

Veggie Tomato Sauce

This is my go-to recipe for all things tomato sauce. With extra veggies and the option to make it in the crockpot or on the stovetop, it's perfect for pasta, pizzas, school lunches, and dipping!

1 tablespoon (15 ml) olive oil

1 red bell pepper, diced

2 medium carrots, chopped

2 medium zucchini, chopped

1 rib celery, diced

1 small onion, diced

2 cloves garlic, minced

½ teaspoon salt

1 tablespoon (16 g) tomato paste

2 cans (28 ounces, or 1.6 kg) tomato purée

1 tablespoon (13 g) sugar

Crockpot directions: Place all ingredients in a crockpot, and cook for 4 to 6 hours on low. Using an immersion blender, purée the sauce, so that no veggie chunks remain. Add water if needed for a lighter sauce consistency.

Stove-top directions: Heat the oil in a saucepan over medium heat. Add the bell pepper, carrots, zucchini, celery, onions, garlic, and salt. Sauté until the veggies are soft, about 5 minutes. Add the tomato paste, and cook for 1 minute more, stirring constantly.

Add the puréed tomatoes and sugar, reduce the heat to low, and simmer for 15 minutes. Remove from the heat, and purée with an immersion hand blender until smooth.

Return the sauce to the heat and simmer until thick, 10 to 20 minutes. For a thicker sauce, simmer for an additional 30 minutes.

YIELD: Approximately 5 cups (1.2 kg)

Kitchen Note

If you don't have an immersion blender, cook the sauce thoroughly and allow it to cool. Mix in your blender (in small batches) so that no chunks remain.

Laura's Tip

Double this batch and freeze the sauce in individual servings.

Homemade O's

Ditch the canned stuff. My homemade version packs a lot more nutrition and is super easy to make.

14 ounces (400 g) pastina, ABC-shape pasta, shells, or macaroni

5 cups (1.2 kg) Veggie Tomato Sauce (page 144)

1 cup (100 g) grated Parmesan cheese, optional

Cook the pasta according to package directions. Mix the pasta and sauce, adding a little water if the sauce is too thick.

Serve in a small bowl and top with the cheese, if using.

For a school lunch: Warm up Homemade O's and place in a warmed thermos container.

YIELD: 8 servings

Kitchen Note

Divide the prepared recipe into individual portions in freezer ziplock bags. Freeze, thaw, and warm when a quick meal or lunch is needed.

Chicken Cordon Bleu Pasta

If you want to score major mom points, be sure to serve this hearty meal for dinner. Not only is this family-size pasta dish a real crowd pleaser, it also yields enough leftovers for a generous serving for lunch the next day.

12 ounces (340 g) penne pasta

2 cups (475 g) Homemade Alfredo Sauce (page 143)

1 chicken breast, cooked and diced

1 cup (150 g) diced cooked ham

6 bacon strips, cooked and chopped

1 tablespoon (12 g) creole seasoning

¼ cup (25 g) grated Parmesan cheese

¼ cup (30 g) shredded Monterey Jack cheese

Cook the pasta according to package directions. Drain, place back in the pot and set aside.

Add the Alfredo sauce, cooked pasta, chicken, ham, bacon, and seasoning to the pot. Stir to combine everything, making sure all ingredients are thoroughly mixed.

Pour the pasta into a 13 × 9-inch (33 × 23 cm) baking dish. Top with the cheeses.

Preheat the oven to broil. Place the baking dish on the oven's middle rack. Broil for 3 to 5 minutes, or until the cheese bubbles and turns light brown.

For a school lunch: Place the warm pasta inside a preheated thermos.

YIELD: 8 servings

Midweek Penne Bake

My family loves this pasta for dinner and anytime in their lunches. Personally, I love the fact that it's so easy to make, I can prepare it with a toddler on my hip! Most of it, anyway.

8 ounces (84 g) penne pasta

1 cup (250 g) part-skim ricotta cheese

2 cups (490 g) marinara sauce

1 cup (150 g) grated mozzarella cheese, divided

½ cup (50 g) grated Parmesan cheese, divided

Cook the pasta according to package directions. Meanwhile, preheat the oven to 350°F (180°C).

In a large mixing bowl, combine the cooked pasta, ricotta, marinara sauce, half of the mozzarella cheese, and half of the Parmesan cheese. Stir to mix well.

Pour into a greased casserole dish, or individual ramekins, and sprinkle evenly with the remaining mozzarella and Parmesan. Bake for 15 to 20 minutes, until the cheese has melted and the sauce is bubbly.

For a school lunch: Reheat the pasta and warm a thermos. Place the pasta in the thermos container and pack inside the lunchbox.

YIELD: 4 servings

Broccoroni

This lunch comes together in about five minutes. It's a great way to quickly put together last night's pasta and leftover broccoli to use.

½ cup (55 g) macaroni pasta, uncooked

½ cup (35 g) broccoli, finely chopped

1 tablespoon (14 g) butter

½ tablespoon (4 g) all-purpose flour

⅓ cup (80 ml) milk

¼ teaspoon salt

¼ teaspoon black pepper

1 tablespoon (8 g) Romano or Parmesan cheese, shredded

Cook the pasta according to the package directions, and drain.

Meanwhile, steam the broccoli until tender-crisp, about 5 minutes, and drain.

In a large saucepan, melt the butter over medium heat and whisk in the flour until smooth. Cook for 1 to 2 minutes on medium-low heat, stirring constantly. When it begins to turn a light golden color, gradually whisk in the milk. Bring the mixture to a boil, and cook while stirring for 2 minutes, or until the sauce thickens. Season with the salt and pepper.

Remove from the heat, and stir in the cheese and broccoli. Toss with the pasta to coat.

For a school lunch: Preheat the thermos and pack warmed Broccoroni, adding a few spoonfuls of warm milk if needed.

YIELD: 2 servings

No Cheese Mac 'n Cheese

I wanted a dairy-free version of mac 'n cheese my youngest could eat and my oldest two wouldn't fuss about. This recipe passed the test! If you don't need to eat dairy-free, feel free to use regular milk.

8 ounces (105 g) macaroni pasta

1 small sweet potato, cooked

1½ teaspoons (6 g) yellow mustard

½ teaspoon ground cumin

¼ teaspoon salt

1 tablespoon (14 g) coconut oil or butter

½ to 1 cup (118 to 236 ml) coconut milk or any unflavored dairy-free milk

Cook the pasta according to the package directions. Meanwhile, cook the sweet potato in the microwave, turning it once, if needed. Peel the potato, and mash it with a fork.

In your blender or food processor, purée the potato, mustard, cumin, and salt to a smooth, creamy consistency. Add a splash of coconut milk, if needed. The sauce will be thick, not runny.

Drain the pasta and put it back in the pot. On low heat, add the coconut oil or butter and mix well. Add the potato purée, and mix until evenly distributed over low heat. Slowly pour the coconut milk into the pot, a little at a time. How much you add depends how much sauce your family likes.

For a school lunch: Heat the pasta and place in a preheated thermos. Add 1 to 2 tablespoons (15 to 30 ml) of milk (or nondairy alternative) when reheating.

YIELD: 4 servings

Zucchini Pasta

My friend, Keeley McGuire, is my go-to for all things gluten- and grain-free. When my kids devoured her zucchini pasta recipe, I knew it had to make its way into this book.

3 zucchini or summer squash

2 tablespoons (30 ml) olive oil

½ teaspoon salt

½ teaspoon lemon peel

1 to 2 tablespoons (2.5 to 5 g) freshly chopped basil

¾ cup (184 g) Veggie Tomato Sauce (page 144)

3 tablespoons (15 g) grated Parmesan cheese

Scrub the zucchini. Remove the ends and julienne by hand or by using a mandoline. Discard the core and the seeds because they do not sauté well in this recipe.

Add the oil to a 10-inch (2.5 cm) skillet over medium-high heat. Once heated, add the zucchini, salt, and lemon peel. Toss over high heat for 2 to 3 minutes, reduce the heat to medium, and cook for 5 to 7 minutes, stirring frequently, until the zucchini is soft.

Add the basil and tomato sauce to the zucchini, toss to coat evenly with the sauce, and remove from the heat. Top with the cheese.

For a school lunch: Make zucchini the night before. In the morning, warm it and pack in a preheated thermos.

YIELD: 3 servings

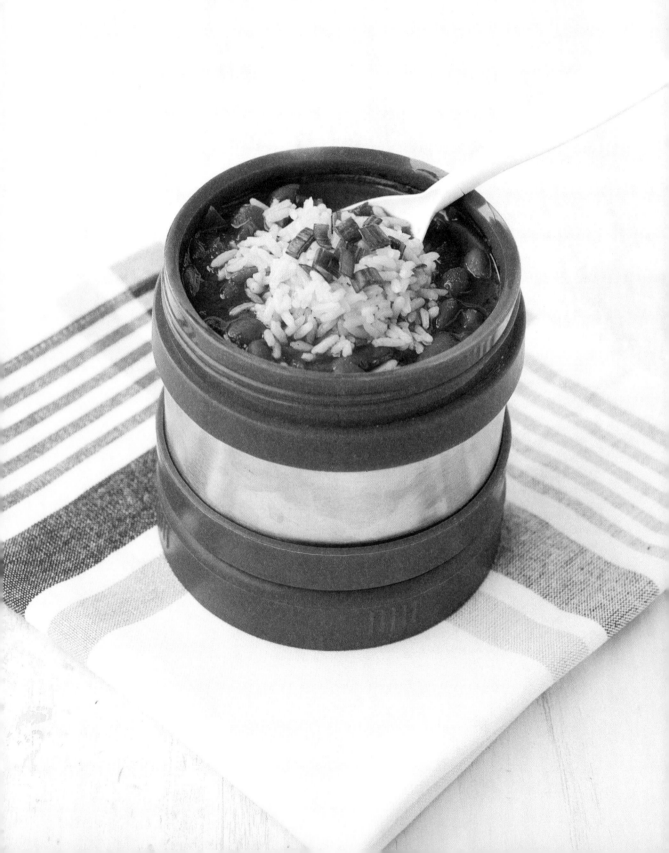

◄ Red Beans and Rice

In New Orleans, you'll find these to be a staple every Monday for lunch, even in school cafeterias. My quick and easy version is delicious and perfect for any thermos lunch.

1 tablespoon (15 ml) olive oil

1 medium onion, diced

2 ribs celery, diced

1 green or red bell pepper, diced

2 cloves garlic, minced

½ pound (220 g) smoked sausage, sliced

1 bay leaf

½ teaspoon dried thyme

½ teaspoon cayenne pepper (optional)

8 ounces (227 g) tomato sauce

¾ cup (175 ml) chicken stock

1 can (15 ounces, or 512 g) kidney beans, rinsed and drained

2 cups (330 g) cooked rice

In a large saucepan, heat the oil over medium heat. Sauté the onion, celery, and bell pepper until they are softened. Add the garlic and the sausage, and sauté for an additional 2 to 3 minutes.

Add the bay leaf, thyme, cayenne pepper, tomato sauce, chicken stock, and beans. Bring to a boil, and simmer for 10 to 15 minutes.

Remove the bay leaf, and serve the bean mixture over the rice.

YIELD: 4 to 6 lunch servings

Dad's Easy Bean Soup

This recipe is the result of my husband's ingenuity. While I was away on a business trip, he realized he needed to come up with a quick lunch, but all that was available was beans, broth, and salsa. So he set out to make an easy soup to fill the kids' thermoses that has now become a family favorite.

1 teaspoon vegetable oil

2 cups (520 g) Homemade Salsa (page 180)

1 teaspoon ground cumin

2 cans (15 ounces, or 864 g) black beans, drained and rinsed

1 can (16 ounces, or 454 g) refried beans

2 cups (475 ml) chicken broth

½ cup (58 g) shredded Cheddar cheese

Heat the oil in a saucepan over medium heat. Add the salsa and cumin, and cook for 3 to 5 minutes or until thickened. Add the black beans, refried beans, and broth; and simmer for 10 minutes.

When the soup is done, fill the thermos, and top with the cheese.

YIELD: 4 servings

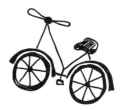

Tomato Veggie Soup

This is the perfect tomato soup to serve with a grilled cheese or homemade cheese crackers.

1 tablespoon (15 ml) olive oil

1 red bell pepper, diced

2 medium carrots, diced

1 zucchini, diced

1 rib celery, diced

1 small onion, diced

2 cloves garlic, minced

1 tablespoon (15 g) tomato paste

3 cans (28 ounces, or 396 g each) crushed tomatoes or tomato purée, with juice

2 cups (470 ml) vegetable stock

Heat the oil in a saucepan over medium heat. Add the bell pepper, carrots, zucchini, celery, onion, and garlic. Sauté until the veggies are soft, about 7 minutes.

Add the tomato paste, and cook for 1 minute more, stirring constantly. Add the tomatoes and vegetable stock, reduce the heat to low, and simmer for 15 minutes.

Remove from the heat, purée in a blender until smooth. Return the soup to the stove, and simmer until thick, 10 to 20 minutes. The longer you simmer this soup, the thicker and more flavorful it will become. You can simmer up to 2 hours. If the soup is too thick for your family, add additional vegetable stock.

YIELD: 6 to 8 servings

White Bean Pumpkin Soup

All of the festive flavors of fall—in one delicious lunch!

1 medium onion, diced

2 cloves garlic, minced

¾ cup (100 g) diced carrots (about 4 carrots)

1 cup (226 g) pumpkin purée

1 can (15 ounces, or 425 g) white beans, drained and rinsed

6 cups (1.4 L) vegetable or chicken stock

1 teaspoon dried oregano

½ teaspoon black pepper

1 tablespoon (15 ml) olive oil

Turn on a crockpot to a medium/low setting. Add all ingredients into your crockpot. Stir to combine. Cook for 4 hours.

You can leave the soup chunky or insert an immersion blender and purée it to a smooth texture.

For a school lunch: Warm the soup in the morning and place in a preheated thermos.

YIELD: 6 servings

Laura's Tip

This recipe freezes very well. Along with some warm whole wheat rolls, this is a fantastic dinner recipe!

Homemade Ramen

In middle school, my cafeteria served a cup of ramen noodles for one dollar. Feeling nostalgic, I worked with my friend Alison to develop this wholesome version.

2 tablespoons (30 ml) extra-virgin olive oil

3 cloves garlic, minced

½ teaspoon ginger, grated (optional)

2 medium carrots, sliced

1 medium leek or 2 or 3 scallions (white part only), cleaned and sliced

4 cups (940 ml) vegetable broth

1 cup (235 ml) water

2 to 3 tablespoons (30 to 45 ml) soy sauce

1 cup (130 g) frozen peas

Kosher salt and pepper to taste

1 pound (435 g) whole wheat angel hair pasta

In a large pot, over medium-high heat, warm the olive oil. Sauté the garlic and ginger, if using, until fragrant. Add the carrots and leek. Continue to sauté until the leeks are translucent.

Add the broth, water, and soy sauce. Bring to a boil, and reduce to a simmer for 5 minutes. Add in the peas, and continue to simmer until the peas are no longer frozen. Season with the salt and pepper.

Meanwhile, in a separate pot, bring water to a boil and add the pasta. Cook until al dente, and drain. The pasta remains separate from the soup to keep it from getting soggy during cooking and storage.

To serve, place a small serving of pasta in a soup bowl, and ladle soup over the pasta. Serve immediately.

For a school lunch: Pack in a preheated thermos.

YIELD: 6 servings

Chicken Taco Soup

My friend Corey has this ability to make just about anything in a crockpot. When she shared this recipe with my family, and everyone devoured it, I knew I had to share it with you!

1 onion, chopped

1 can (15 ounces, or 435 g) chili or pinto beans, rinsed and drained

1 can (15 ounces, or 435 g) black beans, rinsed and drained

1½ cups (195 g) frozen corn

1 can (8 ounces, or 245 g) tomato sauce

2 cans (28 ounces, or 820 g) petite diced tomatoes

1½ cups (355 ml) chicken stock

4 tablespoons (48 g) Arriba! Seasoning (page 106)

1 pound (452 g) boneless, skinless chicken breasts

1 cup (110 g) shredded Cheddar cheese

1 cup (230 g) sour cream

In a crockpot, combine the onion, beans, corn, tomato sauce, tomatoes, and stock. Mix well to combine all ingredients. Add seasoning and stir.

Place the uncooked chicken breasts into the liquid, pressing down until covered by the mixture. Cook on low for 7 hours. Remove the chicken from the crockpot onto a cutting board. Using two forks, shred the chicken and add it back into the pot.

To serve, top bowls with cheese and sour cream.

For a school lunch: Pack in a preheated thermos.

YIELD: 6 servings

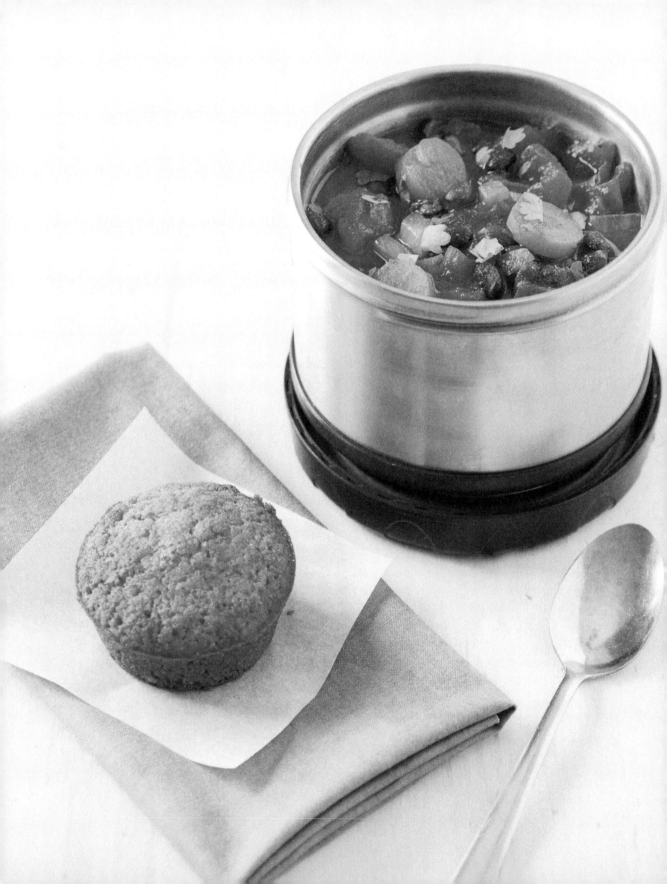

◀ Mexican Soup

With mild, robust flavors, this soup is perfect to fill the thermos on a cold day.

2 tablespoons (30 ml) extra-virgin olive oil

1 cup (130 g) carrots, coarsely diced

½ cup (75 g) green bell pepper, diced

½ cup (80 g) onion, diced

2 small zucchini, chopped

2 cloves garlic, minced

2 teaspoons (14 g) ground cumin

1 teaspoon dried oregano

1 teaspoon chili powder

1 can (14 ounces, or 396 g) petite diced tomatoes, drained

4 cups (940 ml) vegetable broth

1 can (14 ounces, or 400 g) black beans, drained and rinsed

1 cup (235 ml) water

½ cup (95 g) uncooked brown rice

Cilantro for garnish

Heat the oil over medium heat in a large soup pot. Add in the carrots, pepper, onion, zucchini, and garlic. Sauté until just tender, and add in the cumin, oregano, and chili powder. Stir and cook for 1 minute until the spices are fragrant.

Pour in the tomatoes, broth, beans, and water. Cover and simmer for 20 minutes.

Stir in the rice and simmer for an additional 35 minutes. Garnish with cilantro to serve.

YIELD: 6 servings

Tortellini Soup

After you try this soup, you'll never want to eat canned chicken noodle soup again.

2 tablespoons (30 ml) vegetable oil

½ cup (50 g) celery, chopped

½ cup (65 g) carrots, chopped

¼ cup (40 g) onion, chopped

1 clove garlic, minced

¼ teaspoon ground cumin

2 bay leaves

¼ teaspoon black pepper

8 cups (2 L) vegetable stock

10 ounces (283 g) cheese tortellini, uncooked

Freshly grated Parmesan cheese (optional)

In a large pot, heat the oil over medium heat. Add the celery, carrots, onion, garlic, and spices. Cook stirring frequently, for about 7 minutes until the vegetables are tender.

Add the stock, and bring to a boil. Reduce the heat to low, and stir in the tortellini. Cover and simmer for 20 minutes.

Remove the bay leaves. Serve with sprinkled Parmesan, if using.

For a school lunch: Fill a preheated thermos with warmed soup. Serve with Parmesan Crostinis (page 169).

YIELD: 8 servings

Lasagna Soup

This is another "winner" recipe from my friend Corey. After my daughter found this soup in her school thermos one day, she begged for the same lunch every day for nearly a week! Warm, hearty, and satisfying—it's the perfect lunch for a chilly day.

1 can (28 ounces, or 800 g) diced tomatoes, drained

1 can (6 ounces, or 90 g) tomato paste

3 cups (705 ml) beef broth

1 pound (455 g) ground beef

4 or 5 cloves garlic, minced

1 tablespoon (1 g) parsley

1 tablespoon (2 g) dried basil

½ cup (80 g) chopped onion

1 cup (235 ml) vegetable juice (or water)

¼ teaspoon salt

¼ teaspoon black pepper

1 cup (235 ml) water

2 cups (186 g) uncooked shell pasta

1½ cups (173 g) shredded Cheddar cheese

In a crockpot, mix the can of tomatoes and tomato paste. Add broth, ground beef, garlic, parsley, basil, onion, vegetable juice, salt, and pepper.

Cover and cook on low for 7 to 8 hours or on high for 4 to 5 hours.

In the final 30 minutes, add the water and pasta. Stir to combine. Put the lid back on and continue cooking for 30 minutes.

Serve, topped with the cheese.

For a school lunch: Preheat a thermos container and fill with warm soup.

YIELD: 6 servings

Kitchen Notes

Make this soup overnight and put the pasta in the crockpot when you wake in the morning. That way, the entire family will have a hearty, warm lunch.

If you like your soup to have more liquid, add some extra broth or water when you add the noodles.

Lentil Soup

My grandmother made lentil soup like no one else, and this recipe is my best attempt at replicating hers.

2 tablespoons (30 ml) olive oil

1 medium onion, finely chopped

½ cup (65 g) finely chopped carrots

½ cup (60 g) finely chopped celery

1 teaspoon kosher salt

1 pound (384 g) lentils, rinsed

1 can (15 ounces, or 425 g) petite diced tomatoes, drained

8 cups (2 L) vegetable broth

½ teaspoon ground cumin

½ teaspoon black pepper

2 bay leaves

Place the olive oil into a 6-quart (5.7 L) Dutch oven, and set over medium heat. Once hot, add the onion, carrots, celery, and salt, and cook until the onions are translucent and the vegetables are tender, approximately 6 to 7 minutes.

Add the remaining ingredients, and stir to combine. Turn the heat to high, and bring to a boil. Reduce the heat to low, cover and cook at a low simmer until the lentils are tender, approximately 40 minutes. Remove the bay leaves.

Optional: For a creamier consistency, remove 1½ cups (355 ml) of lentil soup and purée in a blender. Pour it back in the pot and mix to combine.

For a school lunch: Pack in a preheated thermos.

YIELD: 8 servings

Ginger Carrots

When my seventeen-month-old devoured these at my in-law's house, I knew we were onto something! Since then, they've become a staple inside his thermos lunches. I typically serve these over Bombay Rice (page 138) or grilled chicken.

1½ pounds (680 g) carrots, peeled and julienned

1 teaspoon apple cider vinegar

3 tablespoons (45 ml) water

1 teaspoon fresh ginger, grated

2 tablespoons (40 g) honey

1 teaspoon ground cinnamon

1 tablespoon (15 ml) olive oil

Salt and pepper

Preheat the oven to 350°F (180°C). Place the carrots in a greased ovenproof casserole dish.

Whisk the vinegar, water, ginger, honey, and cinnamon, and stir the mixture into the carrots.

Drizzle with the oil, and add salt and pepper to taste. Cover the casserole, and bake for 40 minutes.

YIELD: 6 servings

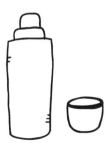

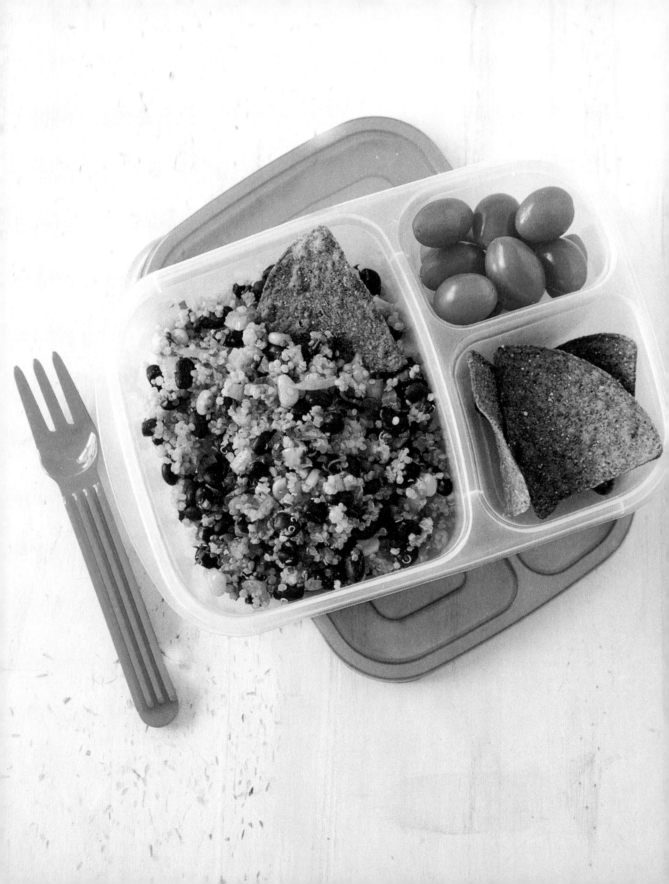

Southwest Quinoa

We weren't big fans of quinoa until we tried it this way. Make this hearty dish part of your lunchbox rotation.

For the Quinoa:

2 cups (475 ml) water

1 cup (173 g) quinoa, rinsed and drained

¾ cup (195 g) jarred salsa

1 teaspoon chipotle chili powder

1 teaspoon ground cumin

¼ cup (4 g) finely chopped cilantro, plus additional for garnish

3 scallions, sliced thinly crossways

1 can (15 ounces, or 425 g) black beans, rinsed and drained

1 cup (130 g) frozen corn

2 medium tomatoes, chopped

For the Dressing:

½ cup (115 g) plain yogurt

1 tablespoon (15 ml) lime juice

1 teaspoon (6 g) salt

½ teaspoon (1 g) freshly ground pepper

1 teaspoon (3 g) garlic powder

Toppings:

1 avocado, diced

1 cup (115 g) shredded Cheddar cheese

To make the quinoa: Bring the water to a boil, then stir in the quinoa, lower the heat, and reduce to a simmer. Cook for 10 minutes, and turn off the heat. Cover and let sit for 6 minutes—you'll know the quinoa is ready when you see the little white "tail" of the germ around the outside edge of each seed.

Once the quinoa is done, add the salsa, chili powder, and cumin, folding to combine well. Mix in cilantro, scallions, beans, corn, and tomatoes. Fold a few times until thoroughly combined.

To make the dressing: In a small bowl, whisk the yogurt, lime juice, salt, pepper, and garlic. Add the dressing, folding gently to combine.

Top with the avocado and cheese, and garnish with additional cilantro.

For a school lunch: Pack the leftovers in a container. This salad is great eaten cold or at room temperature as well.

YIELD: 4 servings

Lunchbox Baked Potato

I don't always have time to make a baked potato in the morning, or remember to make extras at dinnertime! I learned to let the crockpot cook the potatoes overnight, and in the morning, all I have to do is assemble the toppings in the lunchbox!

2 tablespoons (32 g) Homemade Salsa (page 180)

1 tablespoon (15 g) sour cream

1 baking potato, cooked

⅓ cup (58 g) black beans, warm

2 tablespoons (15 g) shredded Cheddar cheese

Pack the salsa and sour cream in small leak-proof containers.

Slice the baked potato in half, top with the black beans and cheese. Store loaded baked potato in a stainless steel lunch container, and wrap the container with a towel to retain the heat.

At lunch, unwrap the potato, fluff with a fork, and top with the salsa and sour cream.

YIELD: 1 serving

Laura's Tip

Cook baked potatoes one night for dinner and make extras. Alternatively, you can bake the potatoes overnight in your crockpot by wrapping each medium potato in foil, and cooking on low for 7 to 8 hours.

Dumplings Lunch

My grocery store deli prepares delicious fresh dumplings. So I thought, why not serve these for lunch? My kids think they are yummy, and I appreciate the time savings.

For the Dumplings:

1 teaspoon oil or nonstick cooking spray

4 to 6 dumplings (also called potstickers)

For the Sauce:

3 tablespoons (45 ml) rice vinegar

3 tablespoons (45 ml) low-sodium soy sauce

1 tablespoon (15 ml) toasted sesame oil

1 tablespoon (20 g) honey

To make the dumplings: In a medium pan, heat the oil over medium heat, and warm the dumplings for 3 to 5 minutes, turning them several times until all sides are golden brown.

Remove from the pan, allow them to cool, and pack them inside a thermos or stainless steel container for better heat retention.

To make the sauce: Mix the sauce ingredients, and pack 1 tablespoon dipping sauce in a small, lidded container. Store extra sauce for future lunches for up to 1 month in the refrigerator.

YIELD: 1 serving

Kitchen Note

If you're using frozen dumplings, follow the package directions to warm.

Mini Tuna Balls

My friend, Keeley McGuire, took the classic tuna salad out for a spin when she created these bite-size yummies. They're a great source of omega-3s and protein, and so delicious, they make lunchtime fun!

1 can (6 ounces, or 170 g) tuna, drained

2 tablespoons (14 g) bread crumbs

1½ tablespoons (23 g) Italian dressing

Preheat the oven to 350°F (180°C).

In a medium bowl, use a fork to combine all the ingredients. Mix thoroughly until the tuna is moistened and smooth enough to roll. With your hands, roll the tuna in about sixteen 1-inch (2.5 cm) balls, then place them on a greased baking sheet.

Bake for 15 to 20 minutes, flipping once halfway through the baking process.

For a school lunch: Serve warm in a thermos or at room temperature in a lunch container. It can also be served skewered.

YIELD: 2 servings, or about 16 to 18 balls

Laura's Tip

Make these the night before. Double, triple, or more the recipe, and freeze the tuna balls after you cook them. For future lunches: thaw, warm, and serve!

Chicken Teriyaki Bowl

This is one of my favorite ways to repurpose leftover chicken and rice from dinner, and my kids love the "take-out" feel and taste of it. Another plus is that this homemade version is far more economical and nutritious than prepackaged frozen chicken bowls, yet offers the same convenience.

½ cup (113 g) shredded cooked chicken

½ cup (195 g) Asian stir-fry vegetable mix, thawed

3 tablespoons (45 g) teriyaki sauce

1¼ cups (210 g) cooked rice

Mix the chicken, vegetables, and teriyaki sauce in a bowl, making sure to toss well to evenly coat.

Over medium heat, warm the stir-fry mixture until thoroughly heated.

Make a bed of warmed cooked rice at bottom of your thermos, or lunch container, and top with the warmed stir-fry mixture.

YIELD: 2 servings

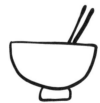

CHAPTER 6

EXTRA CREDIT: STAPLES, DRINKS, TREATS, AND MORE

After helping thousands pack healthier lunches for their kids, I've realized that a great lunch isn't just about the main course. Of equal importance are all the extras that fill the lunchbox.

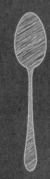

How could I write a homemade lunch cookbook without sharing all of those special extras that help an awesome lunch come together? This section includes my pantry staples, my nontraditional sandwich bread recipes, fun and nutritious smoothies, my go-to dips, and my kids' favorite treats.

Many of the parents in my community find this section the tipping point of going fully homemade. This section will be one of your most visited, guaranteed.

Honey Wheat Biscuits

Wanting to find an alternative to pre-made canned dough, I finally created a recipe my entire family loves. Do not attempt to make this recipe with 100 percent whole wheat flour, or the biscuits will be very dense.

1 cup (125 g) all-purpose flour, plus more for dusting

1 cup (120 g) whole wheat flour

1½ tablespoons (7 g) baking powder

6 tablespoons (85 g) very cold unsalted butter

¼ teaspoon salt (omit if using salted butter)

¾ cup (175 ml) milk + additional for brushing

2 tablespoons (40 g) honey (optional)

Preheat the oven to 425°F (220°C).

In the bowl of your stand mixer, or a large bowl, add the flours and baking powder. Stir together.

Using a cheese grater, shred the butter and add into the bowl. For this reason, I always store a few sticks of butter in the freezer. Using your hands, mix the butter into the flour mixture until it's crumbly and evenly combined.

Form a well in the middle of the dry ingredients, and add the milk and honey, if using. Stir the flour mixture into the milk until a dough forms. Don't overmix.

Sprinkle some flour on your counter and knead the dough. Add additional flour until the dough is no longer sticky. Roll the dough with a rolling pin to about an inch (2.5 cm) thick. Cut the dough with a 2-inch (5 cm) biscuit cutter (or the top of a large glass). After the fourth biscuit, you might need to reshape and roll your dough for the final two biscuits.

Line your baking sheet with parchment paper or a silicone mat. Evenly space the six biscuits on the baking sheet. Brush the tops with milk, and bake for 13 to 15 minutes until a light golden brown.

YIELD: 6 large biscuits

Kitchen Note

You must use a cheese grater for the butter. When I tested this recipe by cutting the butter into very small pieces with a knife, the dough did not rise well, and I had dense spots. Therefore, trust me, and take 20 seconds to grate the very cold butter.

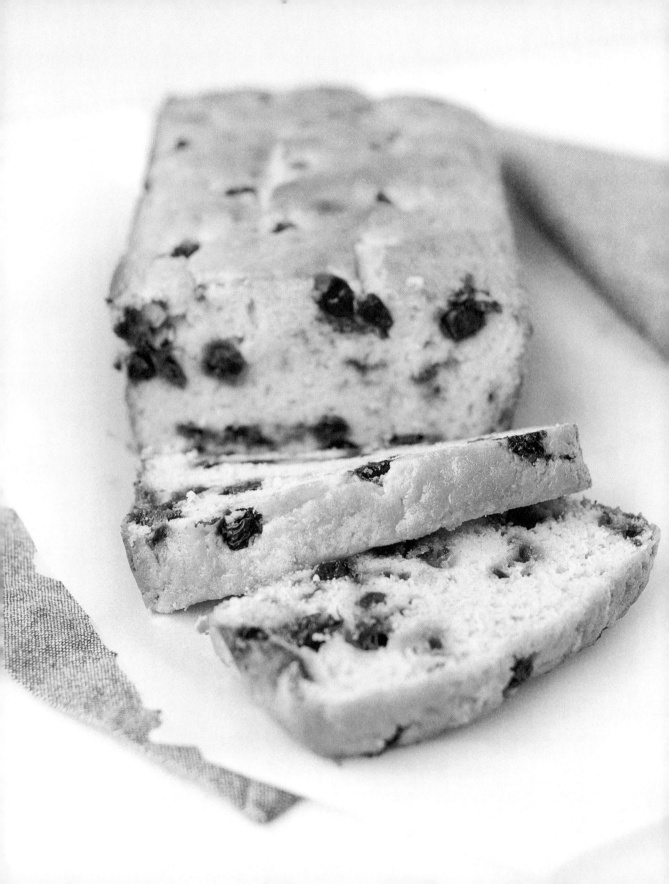

Blueberry Bread

This bread is a staple in our home. The blueberries remind me of warm summer days all year round. Your kids will love it, and soon you'll be making two loaves at once!

1½ cups (218 g) blueberries, fresh or frozen

1½ cups + 1 tablespoon (196 g) all-purpose flour, divided

2 teaspoons (10 g) baking powder

½ teaspoon salt

1 cup (230 g) plain yogurt

1 cup (200 g) sugar

3 large eggs

2 teaspoons (4 g) lemon zest

1 teaspoon vanilla extract

½ cup (120 ml) coconut oil, in liquid form

Preheat the oven to 350°F (180°C). Grease a 9 × 5-inch (23 × 12.7 cm) loaf pan, dust with flour, and tap out the excess. Alternatively, you can line a loaf pan with parchment paper.

In a small bowl, mix the blueberries with 1 tablespoon (8 g) of the flour. Using your hands, toss them around until they are all evenly coated with flour. This helps prevent them from sinking to the bottom of the pan when baking.

In a medium bowl, whisk together the remaining flour, baking powder, and salt.

In a large bowl, or the bowl of your stand mixer, mix the yogurt, sugar, eggs, lemon zest, vanilla, and coconut oil on low speed until all items are thoroughly combined.

Slowly add the flour mix to the wet, making sure there are no lumps, but being careful that you don't overmix. Gently fold the blueberries into the batter. Pour the batter into the pan, and bake 50 to 55 minutes, or until a toothpick comes out clean.

Let the bread cool in the pan for 10 minutes, and then transfer to a wire rack to cool completely before removing from the pan.

YIELD: 1 loaf

Lemon Bread

Sweet and full of lemon flavor, this lemon bread is a household favorite after Sunday service.

For the Bread:

½ cup (112 g) butter

1 cup (200 g) sugar

2 large eggs

½ cup (120 ml) milk

1½ cups (188 g) all-purpose flour

1 teaspoon baking powder

½ teaspoon salt

1½ teaspoons lemon zest

For the Optional Glaze:

1 lemon, juiced

¼ cup (25 g) powdered sugar

Preheat the oven to 350°F (180°C). Grease and flour an 8 × 4-inch (20.3 × 10.2 cm) baking pan.

Cream the butter and sugar in a large bowl. Add the eggs, one at a time, until creamy. Add in the milk, and blend on low speed until combined.

In another bowl, sift the flour, baking powder, and salt. Add the lemon zest and mix. Combine the dry and wet ingredients to create a batter. Pour the batter into the prepared loaf pan. Bake for 50 to 55 minutes, until a toothpick inserted into the center comes out clean. Allow the loaf to cool for 5 minutes prior to transferring to a wire rack to finish cooling.

To make the glaze (optional): Combine the ingredients and spoon evenly over the top of the loaf.

YIELD: 1 loaf

Peanut Butter Bread

I created this bread for my son Alex, who is on the "slim side" and needs all the calories he can get. Luckily, he loves it. It's divine, rich, and nutritious. Perfect for breakfast, or as a sandwich bread alternative.

¾ cup (115 g) brown sugar, unpacked

½ cup (125 g) applesauce

½ cup (130 g) peanut butter

1 egg

1 cup (235 ml) milk

1 teaspoon (3 g) ground cinnamon

1 teaspoon (5 ml) vanilla extract

1¾ cups (218 g) all-purpose flour

1 teaspoon (5 g) baking soda

½ teaspoon salt

Preheat the oven to 350°F (180°C). Grease a rectangular bread loaf pan.

In your stand mixer, or a large bowl, combine the brown sugar, applesauce, peanut butter, egg, milk, cinnamon, and vanilla, and blend until a thick batter forms.

In a small bowl, sift the flour, baking soda, and salt. Slowly add the flour mixture into the wet ingredients.

Bake for 45 to 50 minutes, or until a toothpick inserted into the center comes out clean.

YIELD: 1 loaf

Banana Bread

I often use banana bread for sandwiches to give my picky son a little sandwich bread variety. This is a very basic, no-nuts recipe that my neighbor dropped off on a sticky note along with four overripe bananas. Was it a hint? Probably.

1¾ cup (218 g) all-purpose flour, sifted

1½ teaspoons baking soda

¼ teaspoon salt

½ cup (100 g) sugar

1 teaspoon vanilla extract

¼ cup (56 g) butter, softened

1 large egg

1 cup (225 g) mashed ripe bananas (1 or 2 bananas)

Preheat the oven to 350°F (180°C). Grease an 8 × 4-inch (20.3 × 10.2 cm) loaf pan.

Sift the flour, baking soda, and salt through a sifter or strainer into a large bowl.

In your stand mixer, or a large bowl, combine the sugar, vanilla, and butter, and beat at medium speed until smooth. Add the egg and beat until light in color with a fluffy texture. Add the bananas until thoroughly combined.

Slowly add the flour mixture to the banana mixture, and mix well until a thick batter is formed, but try to not overmix. Pour into the loaf pan, and bake for 40 to 50 minutes, or until a toothpick inserted into the center comes out clean. Cool completely before slicing.

YIELD: 1 loaf

Laura's Tip

You can use up to 1 cup (120 g) of whole wheat flour. Any more than that, and your banana bread will become a banana brick.

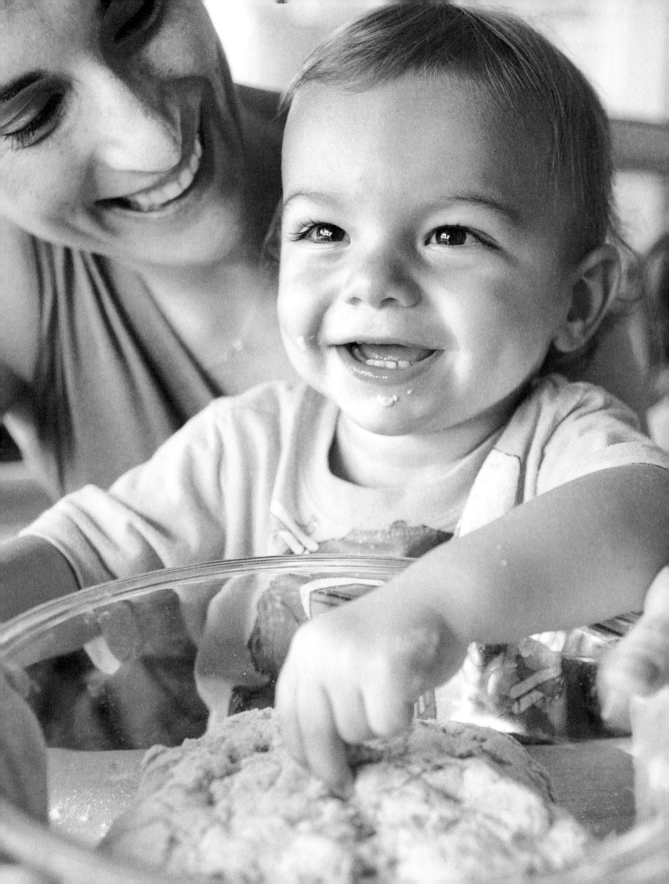

Pizza Dough

Friday night is usually our designated pizza night. This dough is my family's favorite. Lucky for busy parents everywhere, the dough freezes amazingly well. If you want to use whole wheat flour, I wouldn't go more than 50/50 whole wheat to white flour ratio on this pizza. Using additional whole wheat flour will make this a dense dough.

1 cup (235 ml) + 2 tablespoons (30 ml) warm water (120°F [49°C])

1 tablespoon (12 g) active dry yeast

1 tablespoon (20 g) honey

1 tablespoon (15 ml) olive oil

3 cups (375 g) all-purpose flour + additional for dusting

1 teaspoon salt

In a small bowl, combine the water, yeast, honey, and olive oil. Mix with a spoon, and let it sit for about 10 minutes for the yeast to activate. Once you see about 1 to 2 inches (2.5 to 5 cm) of froth, the yeast is done.

In the bowl of your stand mixer, or a large bowl, add the flour and salt. Mix it well. Slowly add the frothy water, and mix it (either with your hands or the paddle attachment) until you can form a dough ball.

Dust the countertop with flour. Place the dough on your countertop, and give it a thorough quick knead. You might need to add a little bit more flour to finish off the dough. The dough shouldn't be super-sticky or rock hard. Good pizza dough should have a "brand new play-dough" or softer consistency.

Rub the same bowl with olive oil, then place the dough inside, and give it a turn or two to coat. Cover it with a towel, and place it in a warm place to rise for about 1 to 1½ hours.

After the dough has risen, transfer it to a floured surface, and knead it a couple of times.

Oil a baking sheet and spread the dough on the sheet to make one large rectangular crust. Or divide the dough into two even portions, and make two smaller crusts. Bake on the sheet at 375°F (190°C) for about 25 minutes.

I like to use my pizza stone in a high-heat/short-cooking time setting. I bake this at 500°F (250°C) for about 10 to 12 minutes. You can, of course, use your stone at 375°F (190°C) for about 25 minutes.

YIELD: 2 medium pizzas or 1 extra large

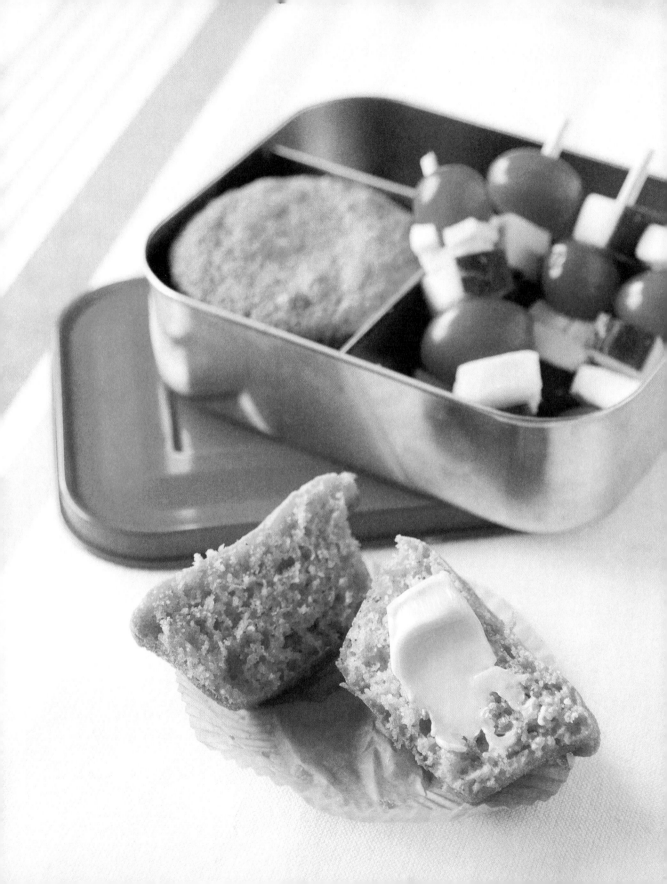

◀ Cornbread Muffins

These cornbread muffins are the perfect addition to the lunchbox! Whether you send them with a thermos full of hearty soup, or as a side with your favorite lunch, your kids will love them.

1 cup (140 g) cornmeal

1 cup (125 g) all-purpose flour

1 tablespoon (15 g) baking powder

½ teaspoon salt

1 cup (235 ml) milk

2 eggs

½ cup (115 g) butter, melted

½ cup (170 g) honey

Preheat the oven to 400°F (200°C).

In a large bowl, mix the cornmeal, flour, baking powder, and salt.

In another bowl, whisk together the milk, eggs, butter, and honey until the liquid is thoroughly combined. Gradually add the wet mixture into the dry ingredients, and stir until just mixed.

Place paper liners in a standard muffin tin. Divide the mixture into the papers, and bake for 15 minutes, until golden.

YIELD: 12 muffins

Parmesan Crostinis

My grandmother used to make these plain, and I improved her wonderful recipe by simply adding a little Parmesan.

1 French baguette, sliced diagonally into ⅓-inch (1 cm) pieces

1 cup (100 g) grated Parmesan cheese (may need additional depending on the size of your baguette)

Preheat the oven to 350°F (180°C).

Place the bread slices on baking sheets. Top the slices with the cheese, and place the baking sheet in the oven. Bake for 15 to 20 minutes, until the bread is crispy and the cheese is golden brown.

YIELD: 18 to 20 crostinis

Easy Freezer Jam

During berry season, I purchase a lot of fresh berries on sale and freeze them for smoothies. Sometimes, I find a bag or two that have been in the back of my freezer a bit too long. But instead of tossing them out, I repurpose them into an easy-to-make jam.

6 cups (780 g) blackberries, raspberries, strawberries, or blueberries

1 lemon, juiced

1½ cups (300 g) sugar

Place all the ingredients into a 5-quart (4.7 L) pot, and bring it to a boil over medium to high heat. Stir occasionally, so the jam doesn't burn.

Bring the mixture to a boil, and simmer for about 10 minutes. Berry jam will begin to thicken. With a spoon, test for thickness, and when you are satisfied, turn off the heat.

Allow the hot jam to cool in the pot to room temperature. Divide the jam into 3 freezer zip bags.

YIELD: 3 cups (960 g)

Cinnamon Raisin Peanut Butter

We love cinnamon raisin everything at our house! And although this might sound a bit odd, this sweet cinnamon-flavored peanut butter tops the charts as one of our favorite spreads. Give it a try, and we're sure you'll love it too!

1 cup (260 g) peanut butter

1 teaspoon ground cinnamon

⅓ cup (48 g) raisins

In a microwave-safe bowl, soften the peanut butter for about 15 seconds. Immediately add the cinnamon and mix well. Fold in the raisins. Store in a glass jar.

YIELD: 1⅓ cups (346.6 g)

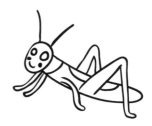

Easy Homemade Chocolate Spread

My kids love chocolate on everything. But when I looked at the store-bought kind and saw that the first ingredient listed was sugar, I knew I had to make my own. And we're so glad I did—this homemade version is creamy, nutty, and delicious!

2 cups (200 g) raw walnuts, toasted

1½ tablespoons (25 ml) vanilla extract

¼ cup (30 g) cocoa powder

¼ cup (60 ml) + 3 tablespoons (45 ml) pure maple syrup (may substitute honey)

¼ teaspoon salt

2 to 3 teaspoons (10 to 15 ml) melted coconut oil or vegetable oil

½ cup (120 ml) coconut milk

In the bowl of a food processor, process the walnuts, stopping intermittently to scrape down the sides of bowl. Continue for 5 minutes until the walnuts have turned to thick, creamy butter.

Add in remaining ingredients, and blend for an additional 4 to 5 minutes, until smooth and creamy.

Refrigerate in an airtight container up to 3 week.

YIELD: 2½ cups (650 g)

Kitchen Note

Feel free to use whatever nut you like, or sunflower or pumpkin seeds. Alternatively, you can use dairy milk, but this will cut shelf life to one week.

Caramel Peanut Butter

This caramel-flavored peanut butter is right on the borderline of being in the treat category. However, every lunchbox needs a little something sweet from time to time. Once you try this, you'll agree. The possibilities for enjoying this creamy, sweet spread are endless!

1 cup (175 g) caramel chips

1 tablespoon (15 ml) maple syrup (optional)

1 cup (260 g) peanut butter

In a double boiler, melt the caramel chips, stirring continuously. Add the maple syrup, if using, as you stir. Once all caramel chips are melted, add the peanut butter, and continue to stir until everything is evenly combined.

Pour the peanut butter into two glass jars. Allow the jars to cool before closing.

YIELD: 1½ cups (390 g)

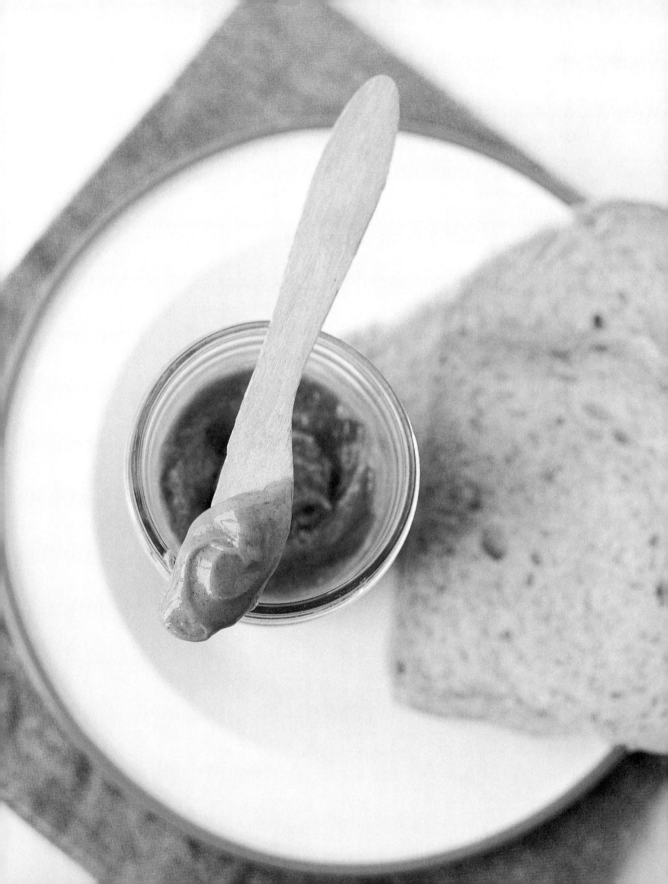

White Chocolate Peanut Butter

My daughter, the chocoholic, who won't eat peanut butter, actually loves this spread. Her imagination of what she will eat and dip into it runs wild every time I make a batch.

1 cup (175 g) white chocolate chips

1 tablespoon (15 ml) maple syrup (optional)

1 cup (260 g) peanut butter

In a double boiler, melt the chocolate chips, stirring continuously. Add the maple syrup, if using, as you stir. Once all the chips are melted, add the peanut butter and continue to stir until everything is evenly combined.

Pour the peanut butter into two glass jars. Allow to cool before closing.

YIELD: 1½ cups (390 g)

Flavored Cream Cheese

Many kids enjoy fruit-flavored cream cheese, but unfortunately the flavor often comes from artificial ingredients rather than real fruit. This recipe provides all the fun and flavor with far more nutritional value!

8 ounces (225 g) cream cheese, softened

½ cup (75 g) strawberries, room temperature

In a food processor or blender, combine the cream cheese and strawberries. Process until smooth and thoroughly mixed.

Store in an airtight container in the refrigerator for up to 10 days.

YIELD: 1¼ cups (281 g)

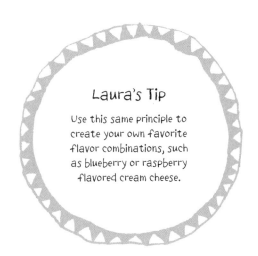

Laura's Tip

Use this same principle to create your own favorite flavor combinations, such as blueberry or raspberry flavored cream cheese.

Homemade Pesto

Packed with vitamin A, healthy fats, and calcium, this easy-to-make sauce brings a lot of flavor and nutrition to any lunch.

2 cups (80 g) fresh basil

¼ cup (25 g) grated Parmesan cheese

¼ cup (25 g) walnuts

1 clove garlic

½ teaspoon salt

¼ cup (59 ml) olive oil

Add all ingredients into a food processor, and purée until smooth.

YIELD: 1 cup (260 g)

Olive Salad

Full of flavor and so easy to make, this olive salad goes great with everything. Over pasta, in sandwiches, in panini's and wraps—the possibilities are endless.

½ cup (80 g) pitted green olives, chopped

½ cup (80 g) pitted kalamata olives, chopped

2 tablespoons (30 ml) olive oil

¼ teaspoon salt

In a large bowl, combine all ingredients. Mix well until the oil evenly coats the olives. Store in an airtight container for up to 10 days.

YIELD: 1 cup (160 g)

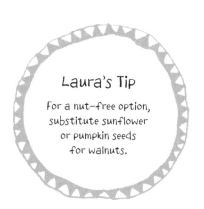

Laura's Tip

For a nut-free option, substitute sunflower or pumpkin seeds for walnuts.

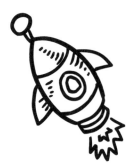

Homemade Ranch Dressing Mix

The only way my daughter will eat raw veggies in her lunch is by dipping them in ranch dressing. Once I realized that I had all the ingredients to make my own, I was happy to not buy the store-bought packets again.

For the Mix:

¼ cup (5 g) fresh parsley, chopped

1½ tablespoons (5 g) dried dill

2 teaspoons (6 g) garlic powder

½ teaspoon black pepper

1 teaspoon dried chives

¼ teaspoon salt

In a small bowl, mix all ingredients together. If you want a fine powder like the seasoning packets, pour all ingredients in a coffee grinder and pulse a couple of times.

To make dressing: Mix 1½ tablespoons (6 g) of the mix with ⅓ cup (77 g) plain Greek yogurt and ⅓ cup (80 ml) milk.

To make dip: Mix 1½ tablespoons (6 g) of the mix with ½ cup (115 g) sour cream or plain Greek yogurt.

YIELD: 4 packets (Each store-bought packet is approximately 1½ tablespoons [6 g])

Greek Hummus

Nobody in my family makes hummus like Yanni. His smooth and creamy version is our favorite for spreading and dipping just about anything! Rich in protein and good for you omega-3s, it's the perfect companion in the lunchbox!

2 cans (14 ounces, or 398 g) chickpeas, drained and rinsed

3 tablespoons (45 ml) lemon juice

2 tablespoons (30 g) tahini

2 tablespoons (30 ml) olive oil

2 teaspoons (5 g) ground cumin

1 to 2 cloves garlic

1 to 1¼ cups (235 to 295 ml) water

Salt and pepper

In a food processor or blender, combine the chickpeas, lemon juice, tahini, oil, cumin, and garlic, and mix for 1 minute.

Begin to thin with the water, adding it in slowly until you reach the thickness/consistency you desire. Season with the salt and pepper to taste. Refrigerate, in an airtight container, for up to 1 week.

For a school lunch: Pack along with fresh veggies for dipping.

YIELD: 2½ cups (284 g)

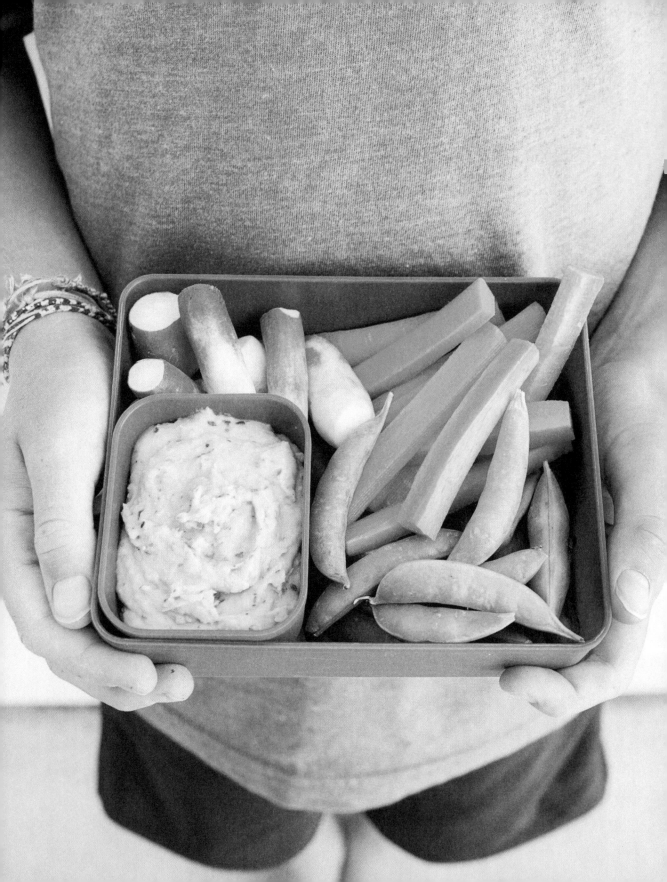

White Bean Dip

Who knew white beans could be this good!

1 can (15 ounces, or 425 g) white beans, drained and rinsed

1 clove garlic

¼ cup (15 g) parsley, loosely packed

2 tablespoons (30 ml) fresh lemon juice

3 tablespoons (45 ml) extra-virgin olive oil

½ teaspoon ground cumin

¼ teaspoon Arriba! Seasoning (page 106)

Place all ingredients in the bowl of a food processor. Pulse until the mixture is coarsely chopped. Pulse a few more times until you achieve the puréed consistency you desire. Transfer to a small bowl.

For a school lunch: Pack along with fresh veggies for dipping.

YIELD: 3 to 4 servings

Greek Yogurt Dip

Full of protein and bold flavor, this dip pairs perfectly with crunchy raw veggies.

½ cup (115 g) plain Greek yogurt

1 tablespoon (15 ml) lemon juice

½ tablespoon (7.5 ml) extra-virgin olive oil

1 clove garlic, minced

½ teaspoon dill, finely chopped

Salt and pepper

In a bowl, mix all ingredients together. Season with the salt and pepper to taste. Refrigerate in an airtight container for up to 3 days.

YIELD: 2 servings

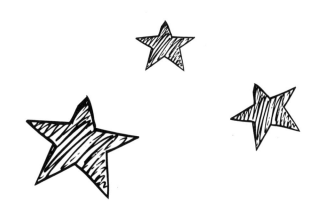

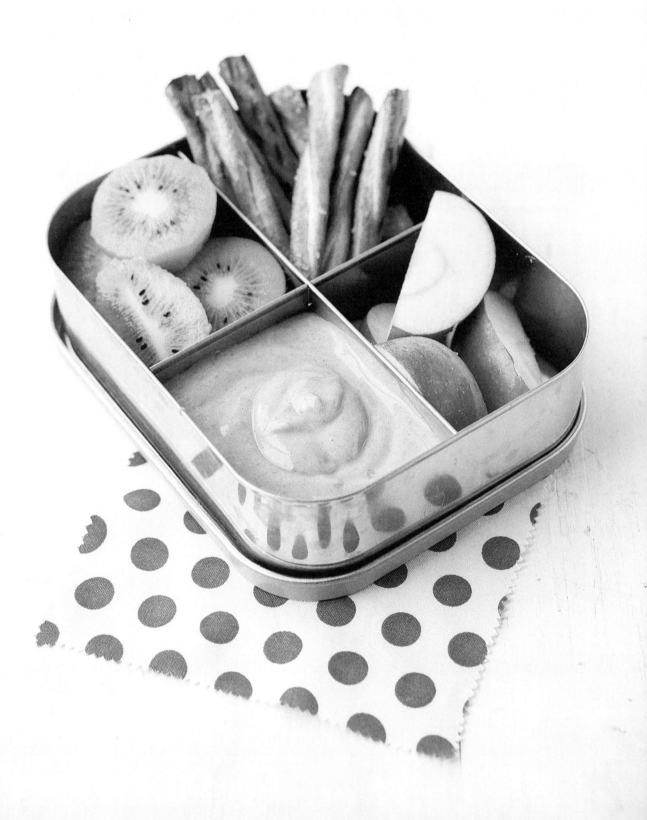

◀ Peanut Butter Fruit Dip

This protein-rich snack will soon become your child's favorite way to eat fruit—or anything else they can find to dip!

½ cup (115 g) vanilla yogurt

2 tablespoons (32 g) natural peanut butter

1 teaspoon maple syrup or honey

In a small bowl, stir together all ingredients until well combined. Serve with your choice of fruit for dipping.

YIELD: 1 serving

Cookie Dough Dip

Perfect to dip fruit or graham crackers—it's high in protein and rich taste!

6 ounces (170 g) vanilla Greek yogurt

1 tablespoon (16 g) almond butter

1 teaspoon maple syrup

2 teaspoons (7 g) mini chocolate chips

In a small bowl, stir together Greek yogurt, almond butter, and maple syrup. Sprinkle with mini chocolate chips and serve.

YIELD: 1 serving

Cinnamon Crunch Dip

This is crunchy and delicious and can be used to dip fruit or eat as a snack.

6 ounces (170 g) vanilla Greek yogurt

1 tablespoon (16 g) almond butter

1 teaspoon maple syrup

¼ teaspoon vanilla extract

¼ teaspoon cinnamon

1 tablespoon (8 g) Lunchbox Granola (page 44)

In a small bowl, stir together all ingredients.

YIELD: 1 serving

Easy Guacamole

Making your own guacamole is so easy, you'll never buy store-bought again. Fresh is definitely better!

2 avocados, peeled, pitted, and meat removed

1 small shallot, minced

1 ripe tomato, diced small

1 lime, juiced

Salt and pepper

In a medium bowl, mash the avocados with a fork. Add the shallot, tomato, and lime juice. Combine well. Add salt and pepper to taste. Chill for half an hour before serving.

YIELD: 1¼ cups (281 g)

Homemade Salsa

So easy to make and far more delicious, you'll wonder why you've been buying the jarred stuff.

1½ cups (270 g) seeded tomatoes, chopped

⅓ cup (5 g) fresh cilantro, chopped

2 cloves garlic, minced

1 small shallot, finely chopped

½ jalapeño, finely chopped (less for a milder salsa)

2 tablespoons (30 ml) lime juice

Salt and pepper

Mix all ingredients in a bowl until well combined. Season with the salt and pepper to taste. Refrigerate overnight for maximum flavor.

YIELD: About 2 cups (520 g)

Kitchen Note

For a thinner and not as chunky salsa, give all the ingredients a few pulses in the food processor.

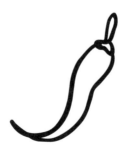

Mango Madness Smoothie

Smoothies are a tasty way to enjoy nutritious fresh fruit. This tropical version is so refreshing—perfect for a warm day!

6 ounces (175 ml) pineapple juice

1 cup (175 g) mango chunks, fresh or frozen

1½ cups (355 ml) ice cubes

Put pineapple juice, mango, and ice in a blender. Blend.

YIELD: 2 servings

The Hulk (Green Smoothie)

It was very hard to convince my son that a green smoothie could taste good. If your child can get past the color, they'll love the flavor.

1 banana

1 cup (235 ml) pineapple juice

½ teaspoon vanilla extract

1½ cups (263 g) frozen mango chunks

2 large handfuls fresh baby spinach

In a blender, combine all ingredients. Blend until smooth.

YIELD: 2 servings

Laura's Tip

Freeze smoothies in plastic freezer jars. Pull them out when you need them or throw them inside a lunch bag in the morning. They will act as an ice-pack and be smoothie consistency by lunch!

Transform Your Smoothie Experience

I love smoothies in the morning, but I don't always have the time to put together a fresh smoothie while getting the kids dressed, fed, and out the door.

My friend, Michelle Castañeda, introduced me to making my own freezer packs, which are essentially just freezer bags filled with ready-to-blend combinations of fruits, or fruits and vegetables.

The concept has revolutionized my smoothie experience, making them convenient, while also completely reducing the amount of fresh produce we waste. For example: I used to purchase a big box of organic baby spinach at the grocery because it was cheaper than the small bag, but half the box would go to waste! Now, when I get home from the store, I put some in freezer bags right away (however much I know we won't be using for our meals), because Michelle taught me that freezing the spinach or other greens has no effect on the taste of the smoothie or on its nutritional value. The same thing goes for my overripe produce. It now goes into my freezer packs, so it's ready for smoothies at a moment's notice!

I've included some of my family's favorite smoothie recipes in this book, most of which can be prepped ahead of time in these packs. (And yes, I am one of those people who reuses her freezer ziplock bags!)

DIY Smoothie Freezer Packs

In a quart-size freezer bag, place dry (that is, nonliquid) smoothie ingredients. Squeeze all the air out of the bag and seal.

Label the bag with the amount of liquid and ice needed. Place the bag in the freezer to keep until ready to use. Servings will vary by recipe.

When you are ready to make smoothies, take the entire smoothie freezer pack and blend with the remaining liquid ingredients until completely smooth.

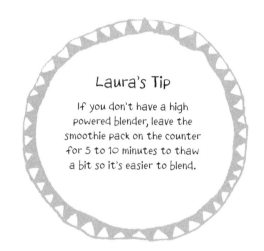

Laura's Tip

If you don't have a high powered blender, leave the smoothie pack on the counter for 5 to 10 minutes to thaw a bit so it's easier to blend.

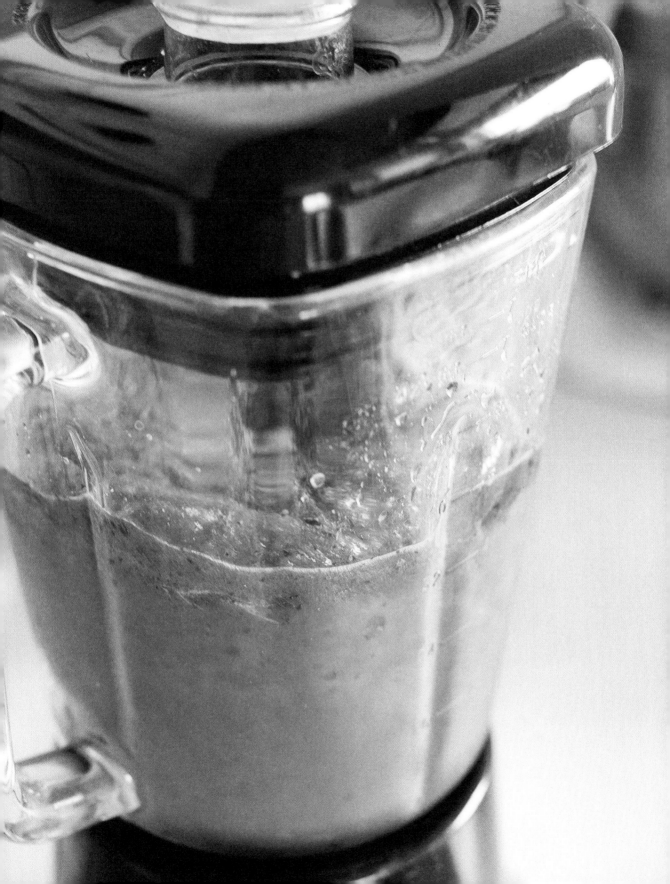

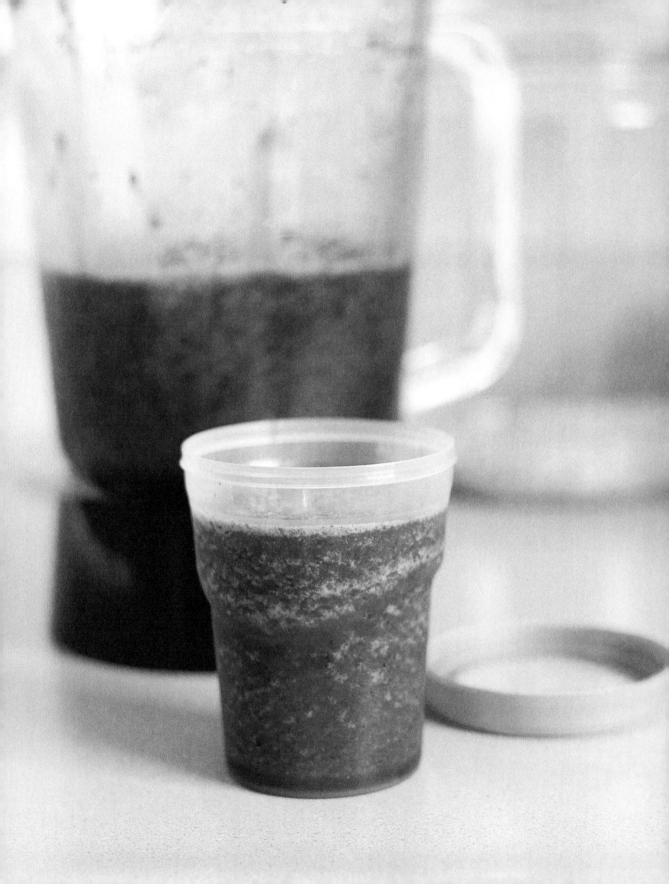

◄ Blueberry Lemonade Smoothie

This refreshing smoothie is perfect to send along with lunch on hot days.

1 cup (155 g) frozen blueberries

1 lemon, juiced

3 tablespoons (45 ml) maple syrup (or honey)

1½ cups (3.5 ml) lemonade

2 cups (475 ml) ice

In a blender, combine the blueberries, lemon juice, maple syrup, and lemonade. Blend well.

Add ice and continue to blend. If it is too thick, add more lemonade or water.

YIELD: 2 servings

Coconut Pie Smoothie

A guilt-free, sugar-free, creamy pleasure rich in coconut flavor!

3 bananas

¼ cup (65 g) cashew butter

1½ cups (354 ml) coconut milk

½ cup (40 g) coconut flakes

1 teaspoon vanilla extract

½ cup (120 ml) ice

In a blender, combine the bananas, cashew butter, coconut milk, coconut flakes, and vanilla.

Blend well. Add ice and blend. If it's too thick, add more coconut milk or water.

YIELD: 4 servings

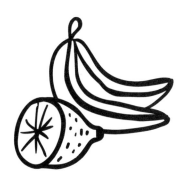

Chocolate Chip Cookie Smoothie

Don't let the "cookie" in the name fool you. This healthy smoothie is both delicious and nutritious.

2 cups (460 g) vanilla yogurt

¼ cup (65 g) cashew butter (or peanut butter)

1½ cups (354 ml) milk

¼ cup (45 g) chocolate chips

1 cup (235 ml) ice

In a blender, combine the yogurt, cashew butter, milk, and chocolate chips. Blend well.

Add ice and continue to blend. If it's too thick, add more milk.

YIELD: 2 servings

Homemade Chocolate Syrup ▶

Real ingredients are what make this chocolate syrup okay in my book. Perfect for making chocolate milk or over your favorite ice cream sundaes. Your kids will never know you made this yourself, and they'll love it just as much.

½ cup (100 g) sugar

1 tablespoon (8 g) unsweetened cocoa powder

2½ teaspoons (7 g) cornstarch

½ cup (120 ml) water

1 teaspoon vanilla extract

In a small saucepan, combine the sugar, cocoa, cornstarch, and water. Over medium-high heat, bring to a boil, and reduce the heat. Stir continuously until thickened to a sauce consistency.

Remove from the heat. Add in the vanilla and stir. Pour into a glass jar and allow it to cool before storing.

To make chocolate milk: Use 1 to 2 spoonfuls of chocolate syrup per glass of milk.

YIELD: ⅔ cup (160 ml) syrup

Kitchen Note

Many nutritionists say that chocolate milk is one of the best post-workout recovery drinks. If you have children who play sports, why not give them a cold glass of chocolate milk when they get home from practice?

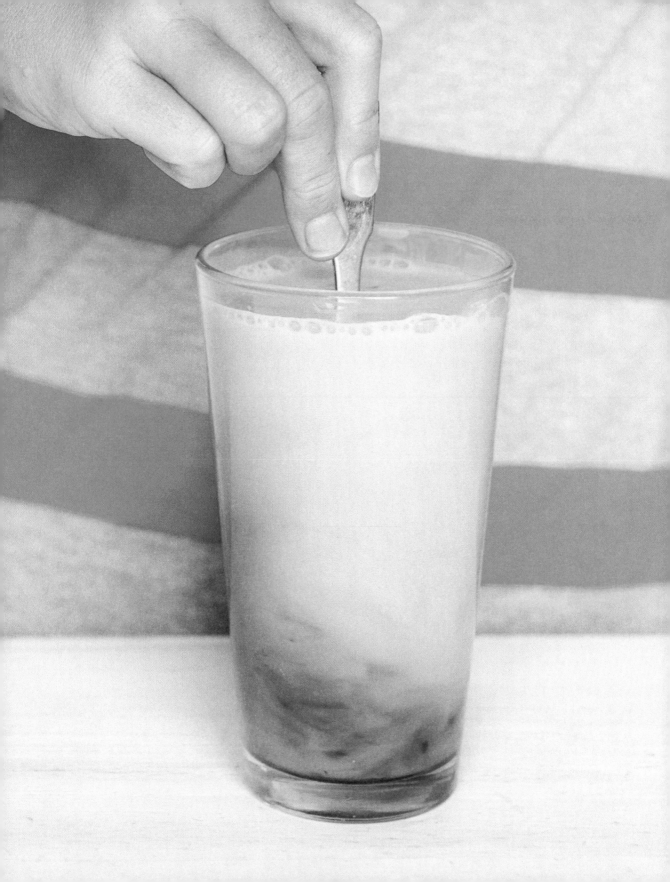

Peanut Butter Cup Smoothie

My son swears this tastes just like the store-bought treat. I'd say even better!

1 cup (235 ml) milk

2 tablespoons (30 ml) Homemade Chocolate Syrup (page 186)

½ cup (115 g) vanilla yogurt

¼ cup (65 g) creamy peanut butter

2 tablespoons (30 ml) maple syrup (or honey)

2 cups (470 ml) ice

Place all ingredients in a blender, and blend until smooth. Add more milk for a thinner consistency if desired.

YIELD: 3 servings

Big Athlete Shake

When our kids need extra calories, it doesn't mean they need to be empty of nutrition. I love this shake because it packs nutrition, it's filling, and it's low in fat—perfect for young athletes and bigger kids with larger appetites.

¼ cup (60 g) plain yogurt

¼ cup (60 ml) milk

¼ cup (38 g) blueberries

½ banana

1 teaspoon vanilla extract

¼ cup (20 g) quick oats

⅓ cup (80 ml) ice, crushed

In a blender, combined the yogurt, milk, blueberries, banana, vanilla, and oats. Blend well.

Add ice and blend.

YIELD: 1 serving

Orange Push-Pop Smoothie

Creamy and tangy are two flavors my daughter loves. This smoothie is perfect for breakfast or packed in a thermos with a school lunch.

½ cup (108 g) orange juice concentrate, slightly thawed

1½ cups (355 ml) coconut milk

½ teaspoon vanilla extract

2 cups (470 ml) ice

In a blender, combine orange juice concentrate, coconut milk, and vanilla. Blend well.

Add the ice and blend. If it is too thick, add more coconut milk or water.

YIELD: 4 servings

Bugs Bunny Smoothie

"Is this what rabbits have for breakfast, Mom?" Yes, of course!

1½ cups (250 g) frozen pineapple chunks

½ cup (65 g) leftover steamed carrots

⅔ cup (160 ml) orange juice

½ banana

¼ cup (120 ml) crushed ice

In a blender, combine pineapple chunks, cooked carrots, orange juice, banana, and ice. Blend well.

YIELD: 2 servings

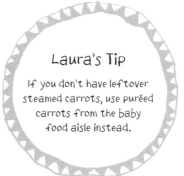

Laura's Tip

If you don't have leftover steamed carrots, use puréed carrots from the baby food aisle instead.

Vitamin C Cubes

These ice cubes flavor the water and add vitamin C. Perfect to help keep those cold bugs away!

One 16-ounce bag (454 g) frozen berries, softened

1½ cups (355 ml) orange juice

¼ cup (60 ml) lemon juice

Add all ingredients in a blender, and blend well. Pour and freeze in ice cube trays.

Place 2 or 3 cubes inside your water container.

YIELD: Approximately 4 cups (940 ml) cubes

Peaches and Cream Smoothie ▶

A tasty way of getting your kids' daily dose of vitamin C.

1 cup (250 g) frozen peaches

1 cup (235 ml) almond milk

2 tablespoons (30 ml) orange juice

½ cup (118 ml) ice

In a blender, combine all ingredients and blend until smooth.

YIELD: 2 servings

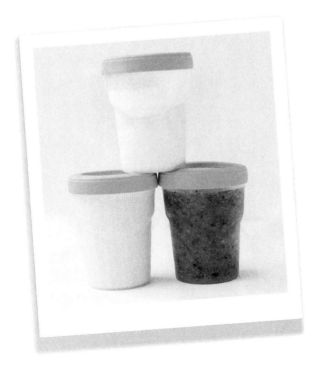

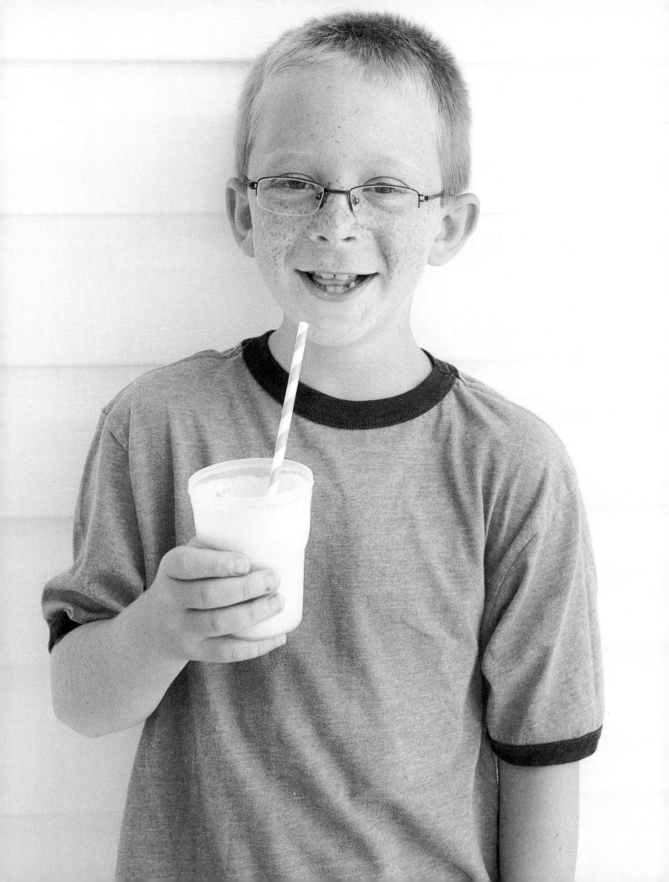

Lunchbox Cheese Crackers

I receive a lot of emails with requests for healthier homemade versions of common packaged snacks to put inside lunchboxes. The cheese crackers one was no exception. This recipe is simple and easy to make, and it will leave you wondering what the extra ingredients in the box are for.

2 cups (240 g) grated white extra-sharp Cheddar cheese

¼ cup (55 g) butter, softened and cut into pieces

1 cup (125 g) flour + more for dusting

½ teaspoon salt

2 to 3 tablespoons (30 to 45 ml) milk

Preheat the oven to 375°F (190°C).

Put everything except the milk in a food processor. Pulse the processor, 5 seconds at a time, about 5 or 6 times, until the dough is in coarse crumbs. Slowly add the milk and process until the dough gathers together into a ball.

Divide the dough into two balls. With a floured rolling pin, roll each dough ball out on a floured surface until it is about ⅛-inch thick. Cut the dough into 1-inch (2.5 cm) squares with a sharp knife or pizza cutter. You can put a bit of flour on the blade of the knife to keep it from sticking. Use a toothpick or skewer to poke a hole in the center of each cracker.

Place the crackers at least ¼ inch apart on parchment paper on a baking sheet.

Bake for 12 to 18 minutes until the edges are just starting to brown. They might puff up too. If you are baking two pans at the same time, swap/rotate the pans halfway through.

Slide the baking sheet off the pan onto a cooling rack, and let the crackers cool completely.

Eat or store in an airtight container or ziplock bag to eat within a few days.

YIELD: 3 to 4 cups

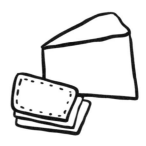

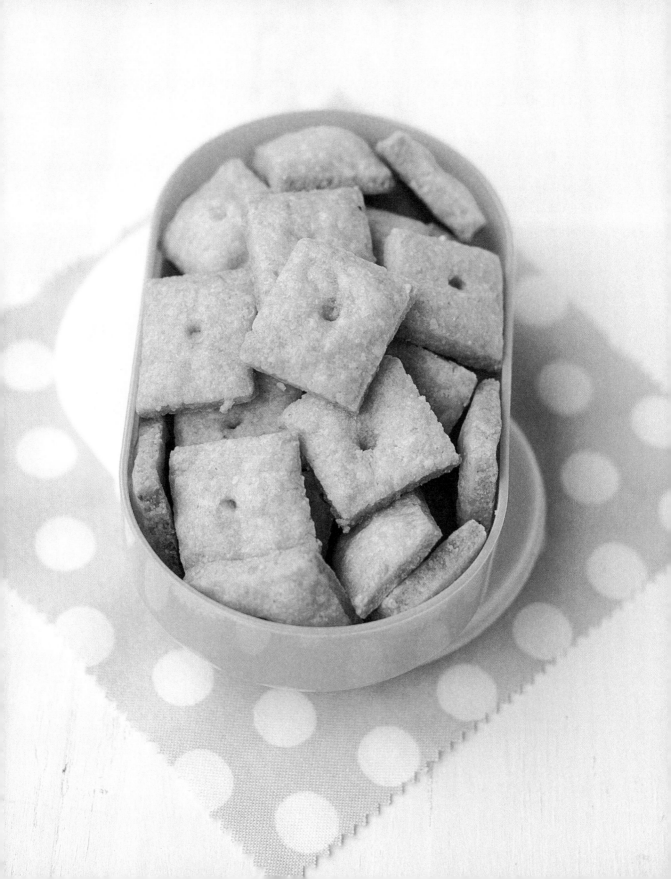

Protein Cookie Bites

My great friend, Kelly Smith, developed these tasty cookie bites. Although we've never met in real life, I think of her each time I pack them in my son's lunch or after-school snack box.

½ cup (130 g) almond butter or peanut butter

¼ cup (85 g) + 1 tablespoon (20 g) raw honey or maple syrup

½ teaspoon vanilla extract

¼ cup (30 g), plus 1 tablespoon (8 g) coconut flour

3 tablespoons (21 g) ground flax seed

¼ teaspoon sea salt

¼ cup (44 g) mini chocolate chips

In a large bowl, mix together the almond butter, honey, and vanilla until creamy and well blended.

In a separate bowl, combine the flour, flaxseed, and salt. Add the dry ingredients to the wet, and mix well to combine. Use your hands to knead the dough. If the dough is too wet, add a bit more flour. If it's too dry and doesn't hold together well, knead in 1 teaspoon (5 ml) of water. Fold in the chips.

Scoop out spoon-size portions and roll into 1-inch (2.5 cm) balls, using your hands to create a bite-size treat. Store in the refrigerator.

YIELD: 18 cookie bites

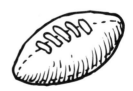

Chocolate Athlete Bars

If you have kids who participate in after-school activities, you know they need extra protein, calories, and nutrition to carry them through the day. Sadly, the best-tasting store-bought bars made with real ingredients are also expensive. Thanks to this recipe, we can ditch that habit and create our own no-bake bars with healthy ingredients—and save a lot of money too!

2 cups (160 g) quick oats

2¼ cups (259 g) blanched almond flour

½ cup (130 g) peanut butter (or any other nut butter)

⅓ cup (115 g) honey

¼ cup (30 g) cocoa powder

1 teaspoon vanilla extract

½ cup (120 ml) milk

In a large bowl, combine the oats and almond flour. Set aside.

In a small saucepan, warm the peanut butter, honey, cocoa powder, vanilla, and milk. Slowly whisk the ingredients so that they melt and combine.

Pour over oat mixture and mix until a thick pasty mix has formed. I find that using your hands works really well to make sure all ingredients are thoroughly combined.

Line a 9 × 9-inch (23 × 23 cm) pan with parchment or waxed paper. Transfer the mix into the pan. Cover with plastic wrap and press down to spread uniformly. Make sure it's well packed down. Refrigerate at least 1 hour, preferably overnight.

Cut into bars or whatever shape you prefer. Store for up to 5 days in fridge or 1 month in the freezer.

YIELD: 10 bars

Kitchen Note

It's important to note that almond meal is not the same as blanched almond flour. Almond meal is ground almonds with the skins left intact, which results in a courser, denser flour with a heavier taste and texture. Blanched almond flour is finely ground almonds with their skins removed, which results in a lighter taste and texture.

Chocolate Chip Date Bars

My friend Alison, the photographer of this book, is an avid runner and mom to three active boys. She needs all the fuel and nutrition she can get from each bite. That's why she loves these delicious and nutritious bars! They not only provide her with a great source of energy, but also make a great snack bar for her boys as well.

1 cup (178 g) pitted dates

½ cup (75 g) peanuts

2 tablespoons (32 g) creamy peanut butter

⅓ cup (60 g) mini chocolate chips

In a food processor, process the dates and peanuts until they begin to form a paste. Add in the peanut butter and continue to process until a dough begins to form. Next, add in the chips and pulse a few times to combine.

Line a 9 × 5-inch (23 × 12.7 cm) loaf pan with parchment paper or plastic wrap, and spoon in the mixture. Press firmly in the loaf pan, until about ¾-inch (2 cm) thick.

Refrigerate for 1 to 2 hours until firm. Lift up the parchment liner, remove from the loaf pan, and cut into 6 bars. Wrap individually and store in the refrigerator for up to a week.

YIELD: 6 bars

Ladybugs ▶

This is one of the simplest snacks, yet kids absolutely love it. Maybe because it's so tasty and adorable!

2 tablespoons (32 g) peanut butter

1 apple, sliced

1 tablespoon (12 g) chocolate chips

Spread the peanut butter onto the apple slices and decorate with chocolate chips.

YIELD: 1 serving

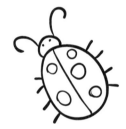

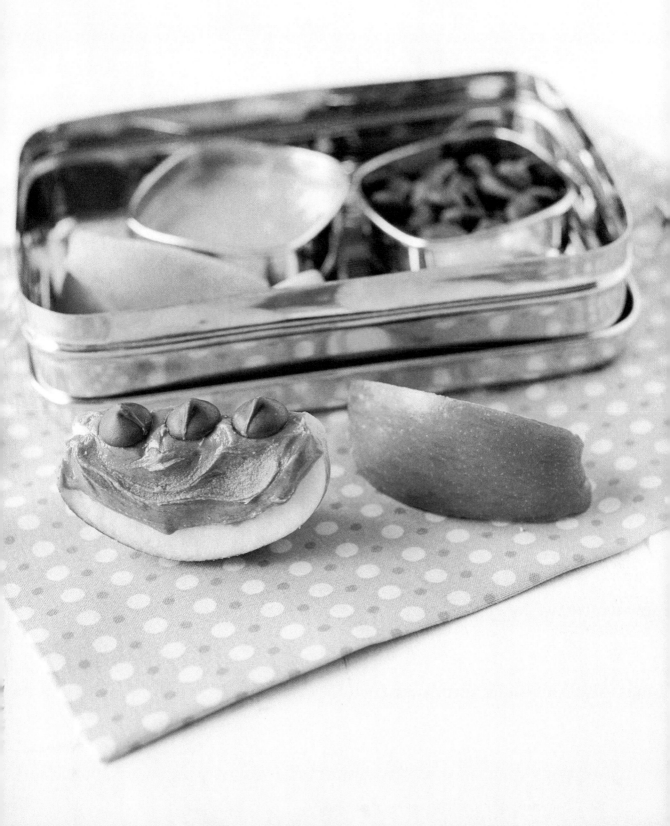

Sweet Ants on a Log

Growing tired of my daughter only eating celery dipped in ranch dressing, I reinvented the classic ants on a log with one of our favorite peanut butter spreads.

¼ cup (64 g) Caramel Peanut Butter (page 171)

2 celery ribs, cut into 3-inch (7.5 cm) pieces

2 tablespoons (18 g) raisins

Spread the peanut butter inside the celery ridges. Sprinkle with the raisins.

YIELD: 2 servings

Maple Glazed Trail Mix

This trail mix is so good, the hardest part about making it is keeping the kids' hands out of it so you actually have something to pack in their lunches.

4 cups (960 g) popped popcorn

2 cups (224 g) pretzel sticks

1 cup (145 g) almonds or pecans, coarsely chopped

½ cup (73 g) raisins

1 tablespoon (14 g) butter

⅓ cup (80 ml) maple syrup

1 teaspoon ground cinnamon

1 teaspoon vanilla extract

Preheat the oven to 250°F (120°C), and line a large baking sheet with parchment paper.

In a large bowl combine the popcorn, pretzels, almonds, and raisins, and set aside.

In a small saucepan, over medium heat, melt the butter. Once butter is melted, add the maple syrup and cinnamon. Stir to combine and heat through. Remove from the heat and stir in the vanilla. Pour over popcorn/pretzel mixture, and quickly toss to coat.

Pour the mix onto the baking sheet and spread evenly. Bake for 45 minutes, stirring halfway through. Allow the mix to cool before serving. Store in an airtight container.

YIELD: 4 servings

Cinnamon Raisin Newtons

My kids don't care for the "crunchy bits" inside fig cookies. For a while, I watched them eat the cookie part and toss out the middle—ridiculous! So, I got creative and made a homemade version with a sweet crunch-free filling that's loaded with important antioxidants.

For the Filling:

1⅓ cups (196 g) raisins

1 tablespoon (20 g) honey

1½ teaspoons ground cinnamon

For the Dough:

½ cup (100 g) sugar or brown sugar

6 tablespoons (85 g) softened butter

1 large egg

1½ teaspoons vanilla extract

1 cup (137 g) all-purpose flour

½ cup (60 g) whole wheat flour

1½ teaspoons baking powder

⅛ teaspoon salt

To make the filling: Place the raisins in a small bowl, and add just enough boiling water to cover them. Let the raisins soak up the moisture for 10 to 15 minutes, until they are plump.

Drain the raisins, and place them in the bowl of a food processor. Add the honey and cinnamon and purée the mixture until it is a smooth paste.

To make the dough: Preheat the oven to 350°F (180°C).

In the bowl of a stand mixer, or a large bowl, cream the sugar and butter until smooth. Add the egg and vanilla, and mix for another 2 minutes until it becomes a sweet paste.

In a small bowl, combine the flours, baking powder, and salt. Gradually add the flour mixture into the sugar mixture, on low speed, until a dough forms. Remove the dough from the bowl, give it a quick hand knead and divide it in two pieces.

Roll the first dough piece between two pieces of parchment paper into a 12 × 4-inch (30 × 10 cm) rectangle. Remove the top piece of paper. Spread half of the cinnamon raisin paste along the center third of the rectangle nearly all the way to the top and bottom edges.

Using the bottom piece of parchment paper to assist you, lift one-third of the dough rectangle and put it on top of half of the raisin paste. Repeat the process with the other side, and gently press the dough along the center line and top and bottom edges. Repeat the process with the second half of the dough.

Cut each rectangular log into 8 to 10 pieces. Transfer to a parchment paper–lined baking sheet. Bake for 18 minutes, or until golden brown. Allow the cookies to cool before serving, and store in an airtight container for up to 5 days.

YIELD: 18 to 20 cookies

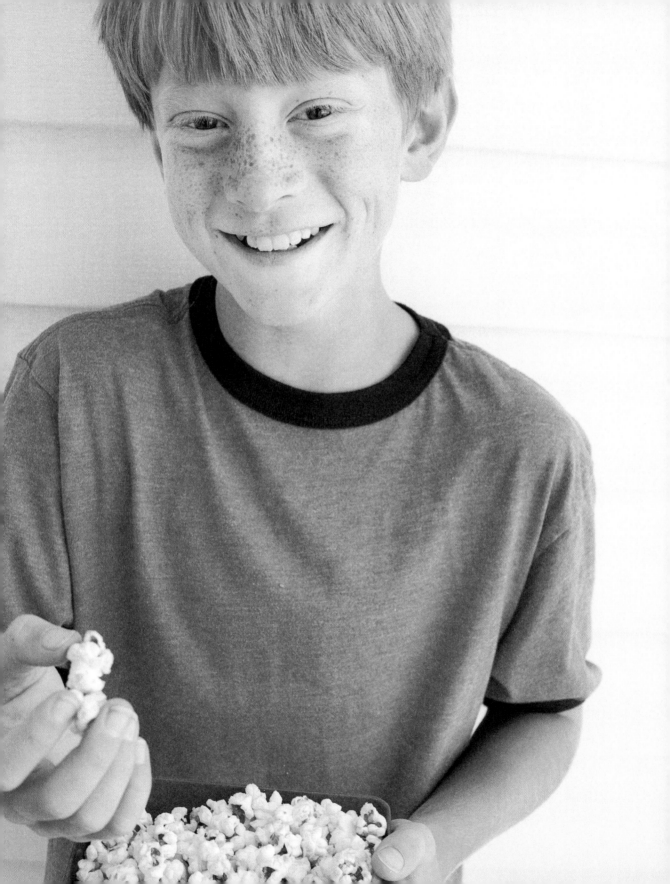

Kettle Corn

Kettle corn is the perfect snack for kids who crave a little sweetness in their lunchbox. It's also the perfect treat for movie night!

3 tablespoons (45 ml) vegetable oil

1 cup (200 g) popcorn kernels

⅓ cup (150 g) granulated sugar

½ teaspoon kosher salt

Heat a large, heavy bottomed pot (soup or stockpot) over medium-high heat. Add the vegetable oil to the pot and allow it to get hot.

Add the popcorn kernels, and stir until all are coated with the oil. When the kernels begin to pop, stir in the sugar. Cover the pot with a lid, and occasionally shake it to move kernels around and prevent burning.

When the popping slows, remove from the stovetop and pour the popcorn onto parchment paper. Spread into a single layer, and sprinkle with the salt. Allow the popcorn to cool before eating.

YIELD: 4 servings

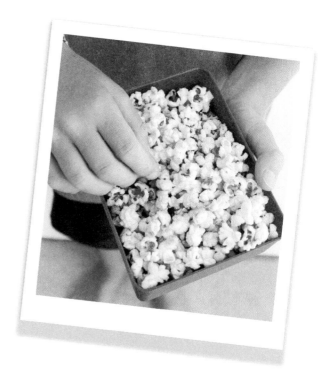

Caramel Banilla Bites

When my friend Corey Valley told me about Banilla bites, I thought she was a genius! I've changed her recipe so that it uses my caramel peanut butter and boy, oh boy, are these delicious!

⅓ cup (87 g) Caramel Peanut Butter (page 171)

12 round vanilla wafers

1 banana, sliced into 6 thick pieces

Colored sprinkles, optional

Spread a small amount of peanut butter onto each wafer. Place a slice of banana in the middle of 6 wafers, and top with remaining wafers.

Place sprinkles, if using, in a shallow bowl, and roll the cookies over the sprinkles a couple of times until the sides are covered.

YIELD: 6 servings

Rainbow Fruit Cups ▶

This is the perfect way of making fruit portable, convenient, and slightly sweet without the unhealthy additives and sugars found in the packaged ones.

2 kiwis, peeled and cut into large chunks

1 cup (125 g) raspberries

1 cup (145 g) blueberries

1 tablespoon (20 g) maple syrup

In a large bowl, combine the fruit and maple syrup. Toss well to evenly coat.

Distribute evenly among 4 small leak-proof containers.

YIELD: 4 servings

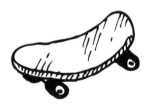

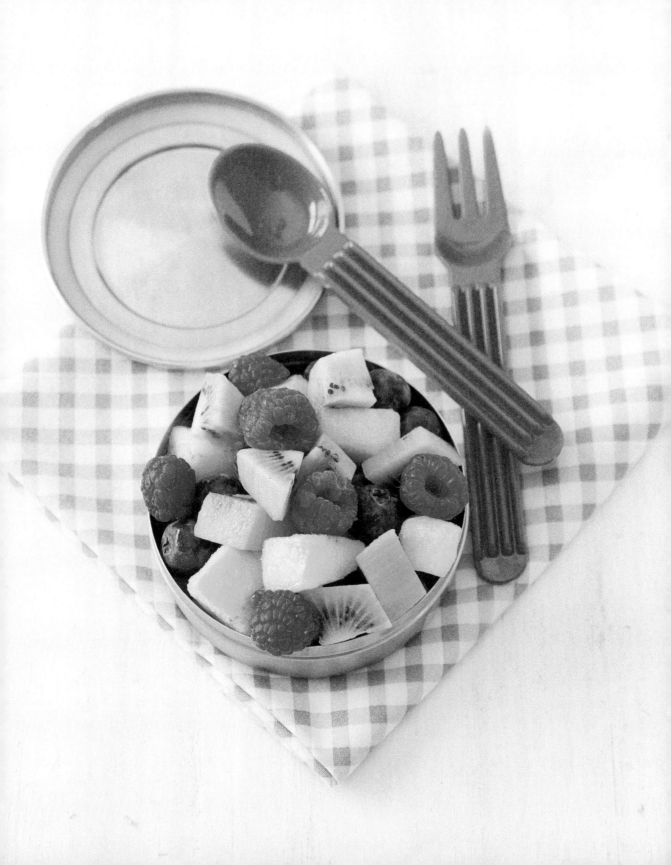

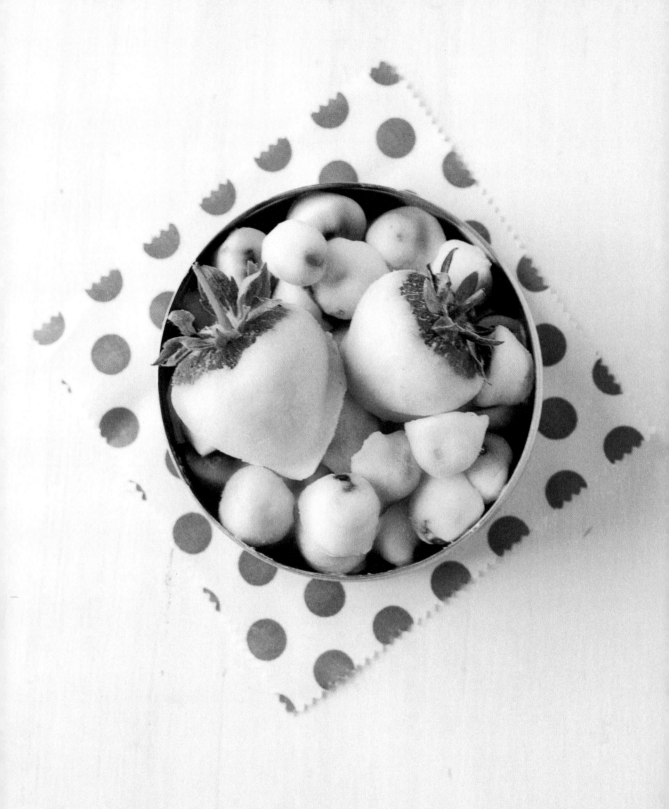

◀ Frozen Yogurt Berries

Each sweet bite carries a little protein and vitamin C. It's the perfect afterschool snack!

6 ounces (145 g) fresh blueberries, washed

12 ounces (345 g) vanilla Greek yogurt

1 cup (145 g) fresh strawberries, washed

Line a baking sheet with parchment paper.

Using a toothpick, dip each blueberry into the yogurt and swirl until the blueberry is nicely coated with yogurt. Place on the baking sheet. Continue until all the blueberries are coated.

Dip the strawberries into the yogurt halfway up and lay on the baking sheet. Place the baking sheet into the freezer for at least an hour.

The strawberries should be consumed after an hour of freezing for the best flavor. Place any leftover strawberries in a ziplock bag and freeze for use in smoothies. The blueberries can be placed in a ziplock baggie and stored in the freezer. Take out what you need for snack time and enjoy!

YIELD: 6 servings, or 3 cups

No-Bake Brownie Bites

These bite-size treats are the perfect brain food! Loaded with antioxidants, protein, and vitamins, they pack a nutritional punch in every yummy bite.

½ cup (73 g) raisins

1 cup (235 ml) boiling water

⅓ cup (114 g) honey

2 teaspoons (30 ml) vanilla extract

1¾ cups (198 g) almond flour

3 tablespoons (41 g) unsweetened cocoa powder

⅓ cup (58 g) mini chocolate chips

Place the raisins in a small bowl, and pour the water over to cover. Allow the raisins to plump up for about 10 minutes, then drain and put the raisins in your food processor bowl.

Add the honey and vanilla to the bowl, and process until a thick paste forms. Add the flour and cocoa powder, and process until a dough has formed.

Transfer the dough into a bowl, fold in the chips, and refrigerate for 10 minutes. By doing this, the dough will be easier to shape. Once ready, use your hands to form and roll into bite-size balls. Refrigerate until ready to eat.

YIELD: 12 brownie bites

Kitchen Note

Store brownie bites in the freezer for up to 3 months. For a lunchbox treat, stick them in the lunchbox frozen. They will thaw by lunchtime.

Oatmeal Raisin Granola Bars

My daughter loves granola bars. The problem is that the organic ones she likes are quite expensive! My sweet girl tested dozens of not-so-good chewy recipes until I finally came up with one she loved. At my house, we call these Sofia Bars.

2 cups (160 g) quick oats

1 cup (200 g) crispy rice cereal

⅛ teaspoon salt

3 heaping tablespoons (27 g) raisins

¼ cup (55 g) butter or coconut oil

¼ cup (60 ml) brown rice syrup

¼ cup (60 g) brown sugar, packed

1 teaspoon vanilla extract

Line an 8 × 8-inch (20.3 × 20.3 cm) or 9 × 9-inch (23 × 23 cm) baking pan or glass baking dish with parchment paper. In a large bowl, mix the oats, cereal, salt, and raisins. Set aside.

In a small pot, melt the butter, syrup, and brown sugar. When it starts to boil, reduce the heat to medium-low, and cook for 4 minutes, making sure the mixture continues to minimally bubble while stirring often. Turn off the heat and add the vanilla.

Pour the liquid mixture into the dry ingredients, and mix well to combine all ingredients. Place the mixture into the baking dish. Cover with parchment paper, and press down with your hands until the mix is well packed. (Just when you think you've pressed down enough—press some more!)

Allow the pan to cool at room temperature for at least 2 hours. Lift parchment paper out onto a cutting board and slice into 12 bars. After cutting the bars, store in an airtight container or ziplock bag for up to 1 week.

YIELD: 12 bars

Kitchen Note

You can find brown rice syrup in the baking aisle of your health-food store and online. Alternatively, you could use honey, but the bars will be sticky and they tend to break apart easier, which is why I don't recommend using it.

Laura's Tip

Want to make these chocolate chip bars instead? Omit the raisins and wait until mixture has cooled 30 minutes on the pressed pan. Then sprinkle with chocolate chips and press down again to add them to the bars.

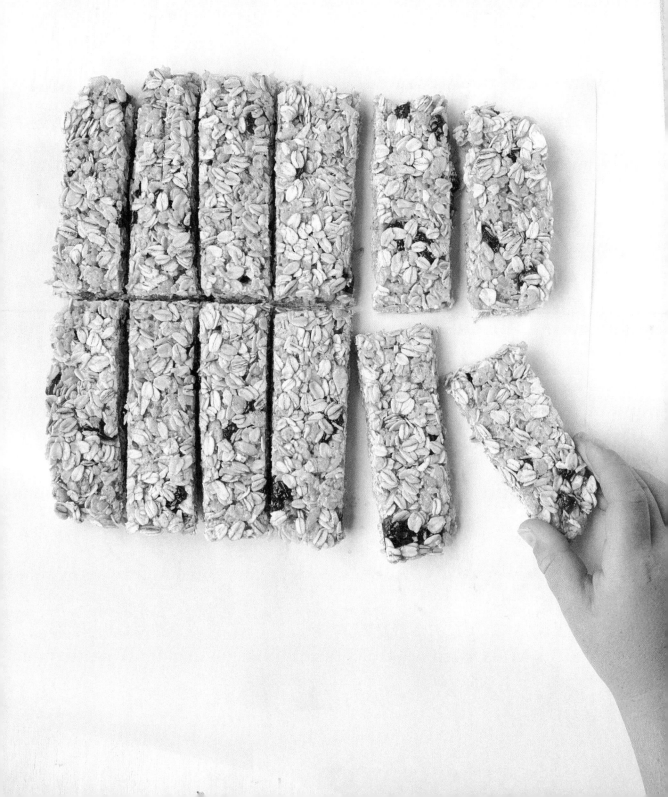

Strawberry Shortcake Kabobs

I love assembling a tray of these shortcake kabobs and keeping them in the fridge for play dates, an easy lunchbox treat, or lazy afternoon snack.

1 loaf Lemon Bread (page 164)

1 pound (510 g) fresh strawberries, whole or halved

½ cup (88 g) milk chocolate chips

½ cup (88 g) white chocolate chips

Slice the bread into ¾-inch (2 cm) thick slices. Cut into vertical strips, then into cubes.

Alternate skewering the bread cubes and strawberries through small wooden sticks. Once assembled, lay them flat on a baking sheet.

In the microwave, melt both milk chocolate and white chocolate chips in separate containers, making sure you stir every 15 seconds so that the chocolate doesn't burn.

Drizzle the melted white chocolate and milk chocolate over the kabobs. Allow the chocolate to cool, transfer the tray into the refrigerator, and store until ready to serve.

YIELD: 12 to 18 skewers

White Chocolate Peanut Butter Strawberry Crostinis ▶

When my friend Alison emailed me to tell me that her boys begged for these as their afternoon snack, I knew they were cookbook-worthy.

4 plain crostinis

2 tablespoons (32 g) White Chocolate Peanut Butter (page 173)

2 large strawberries, sliced

Make plain crostinis from the Parmesan Crostinis recipe on page 169 by omitting Parmesan cheese.

Spread the peanut butter onto the crostinis. Top with the strawberry slices.

YIELD: 1 serving

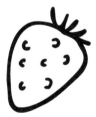

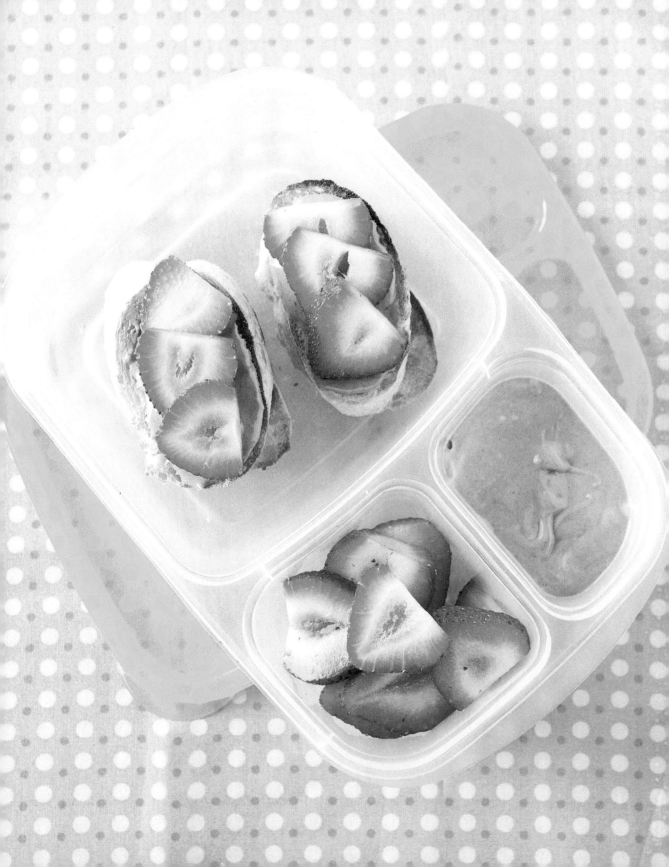

Banana Split Bites

Ditch the boxed chocolate cookies, ice cream, and whipped toppings. Most are full of unidentifiable ingredients and very little nutrition. These sweet pieces of frozen fruit encased in chocolate shells are the perfect after-school snack your kids will love!

Twelve 1-inch (2.5 cm) pieces fresh pineapple

1 under-ripe banana, cut into ½-inch (1.3 cm) slices

6 medium strawberries, sliced in half

⅓ cup (58 g) dark chocolate chunks

1 teaspoon coconut oil

Chopped nuts or shredded coconut (optional), for decoration

Line a baking sheet with parchment paper. Press a small wooden stick through each piece of fruit and freeze until solid (for about 1 hour) on the baking sheet.

Melt the chocolate along with the coconut oil in a double broiler on the stove or in the microwave, stirring frequently (every 15 to 20 seconds) to prevent burning. Once the chocolate is completely melted, remove the frozen fruit from the freezer.

Dip the fruit in the chocolate, let the excess drip off, and place back on the sheet while it hardens. If using, dip the chocolate-covered side immediately in chopped nuts or coconut before placing them on the sheet to harden.

Once the chocolate is completely hardened, remove from the sheet, and place in an airtight container to store in the freezer until ready to serve.

YIELD: 12 banana split bites

Kitchen Note

If you use a ripe banana, the sugars break down, which will result in a mushy banana once thawed.

Laura's Tip

Keep these in the freezer in an airtight container or ziplock bag for when the kids get home from school.

Flourless Chocolate Cookies

My husband packs an extra cookie or two in all of our lunchboxes when these are around. He rationalizes that since they have flaxseed, they must be good. And he's not far off track, since flaxseed is a great source of fiber and omega-3s.

1 cup (260 g) peanut butter

1 cup (225 g) brown sugar, packed

1 large egg

1½ teaspoons vanilla extract

2 tablespoons (30 ml) water

⅓ cup (40 g) cocoa powder

¼ cup (42 g) finely ground flaxseed

1½ teaspoons baking soda

In a medium bowl, mix the peanut butter, brown sugar, egg, vanilla, and water until thoroughly combined.

Slowly add the cocoa powder, flaxseed, and baking soda. Mix on low speed until all the cocoa has been incorporated into the mixture and there are no clumps.

Transfer the dough to an airtight container, and refrigerate for 1 hour or up to 5 days. When ready to bake, preheat the oven to 350°F (180°C).

Line two baking sheets with parchment paper. Scoop golf ball–size dough mounds onto the baking sheets at least 2 inches (5 cm) apart.

Bake for 10 minutes, until the edges are set in shape, even if the middle seems a little gooey, making sure to switch the tray's position about halfway through. Cookies will harden and set as they cool. Once they are no longer hot, transfer to racks to finish cooling.

YIELD: 24 cookies

Halloween Loot Cookies

Swapping out chocolate chips for leftover chocolate Halloween candy will help you get through the loot a little quicker, and not in one sitting.

2¼ cups (282 g) all-purpose flour

1 teaspoon baking soda

1 teaspoon salt

1 cup (225 g) butter, softened

¾ cup (150 g) granulated sugar

¾ cup (170 g) packed brown sugar

1 teaspoon vanilla extract

2 large eggs

2 cups (350 g) chocolate Halloween candy, chopped

Preheat the oven to 375°F (190°C). Line two baking sheets with parchment paper.

Combine the flour, baking soda, and salt in a bowl. In a large mixer bowl, beat the butter, sugars, and vanilla until creamy. Add the eggs, one at a time, beating well after each addition. Gradually beat in the flour mixture. Fold in the candy.

Spoon golf ball–size dough balls onto lined baking sheets. Bake for 9 to 11 minutes or until golden brown. Cool on the baking sheets for 2 minutes; remove to wire racks to cool completely.

YIELD: 24 cookies

White Chocolate Chip Cookies ▶

Chocolate chip cookies are a lunchbox classic. This white chip version is a favorite with my kids, and I prefer them because they don't get their school clothes messy!

2¼ cups (282 g) all-purpose flour

1 teaspoon baking soda

1 teaspoon salt

1 cup (225 g) (2 sticks) butter, softened

¾ cup (200 g) granulated sugar

¾ cup (170 g) packed brown sugar

1 teaspoon vanilla extract

2 large eggs

2 cups (350 g) white chocolate chips

Preheat the oven to 375°F (190°C).

In a small bowl, combine the flour, baking soda, and salt. In a large mixer bowl, beat the butter, granulated sugar, brown sugar, and vanilla until creamy. Add the eggs, one at a time, beating well after each addition.

Gradually beat in the flour mixture. Stir in the chips. Drop by rounded tablespoon onto ungreased baking sheets.

Bake for 9 to 11 minutes or until golden brown. Cool on baking sheets for 2 minutes; remove to wire racks to cool completely.

YIELD: 4 dozen cookies

Kitchen Note

Make extra batches of the cookie dough, and freeze single-portioned cookie dough balls for future baking.

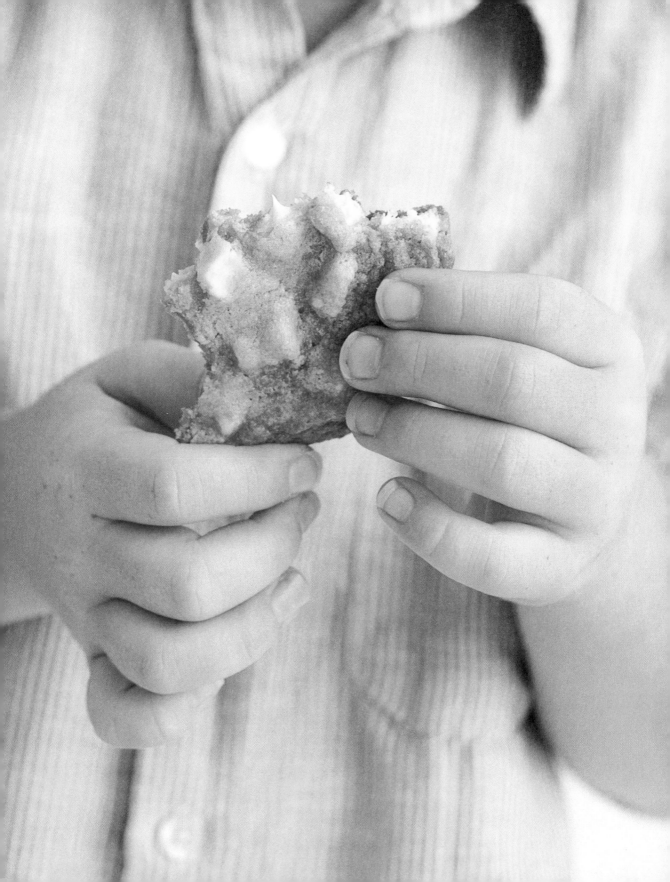

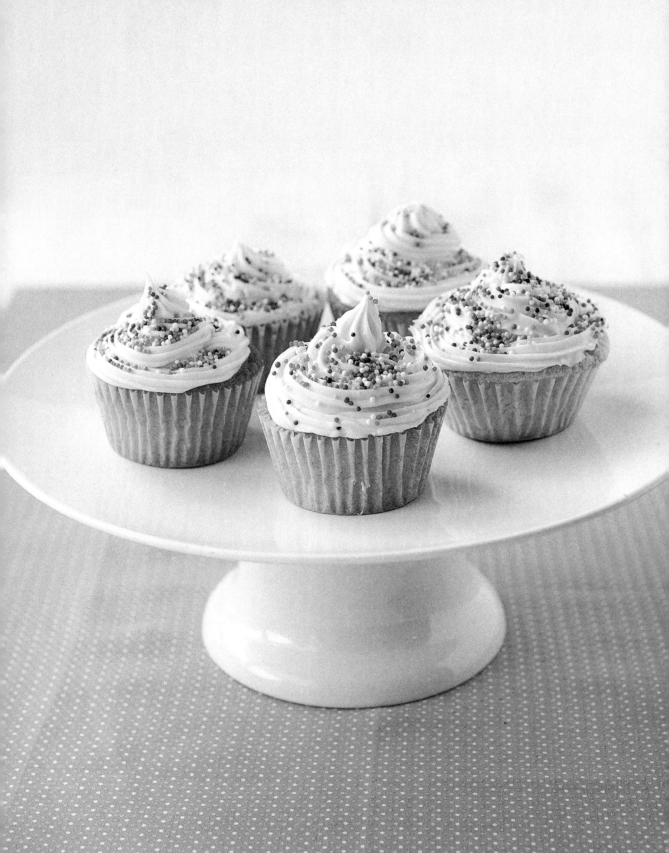

Classroom Cupcakes

This recipe, adapted from *Cooks Illustrated* to make the process easier, became what I call a one-bowl wonder. It uses ingredients readily available in your pantry and comes together quicker than you can go to the store to purchase a box of cake mix.

For the Cupcakes:

1½ cups (188 g) all-purpose flour, sifted

1 cup (200 g) granulated sugar

1½ teaspoons baking powder

½ teaspoon salt

8 tablespoons (112 g) unsalted butter, room temperature

½ cup (115 g) Greek yogurt

2 large eggs, room temperature

1½ teaspoons vanilla extract

For the Frosting:

3 cups (300 g) powdered sugar

1 cup (448 g) butter, softened

1 teaspoon vanilla extract

1 to 2 tablespoons (15 to 30 ml) heavy cream

Adjust the oven rack to the middle position. Preheat the oven to 350° F (180°C). Line a standard cupcake pan with paper liners.

To make the cupcakes: In the bowl of your standing mixer, mix the flour, sugar, baking powder, and salt. Add the butter, yogurt, eggs, and vanilla, and beat at medium speed until smooth, about 30 seconds. Scrape down the sides of the bowl with a rubber spatula, and mix by hand until smooth and no flour pockets remain.

Divide the thick batter evenly among the cups (about two-thirds full) of the prepared tin. I like to use an ice cream scoop for this. Bake until the cupcake tops are pale gold and a toothpick inserted into the center comes out clean, about 22 minutes.

Remove from the oven; allow to cool for 5 minutes before removing the cupcakes from the tin and transferring to a wire rack. Cool the cupcakes to room temperature before frosting.

To make the frosting: In a large bowl, whisk the sugar and butter on low speed until well blended. Increase speed to medium, and beat for an additional 3 minutes.

Add the vanilla and cream, and beat on medium speed for 1 minute.

YIELD: 12 cupcakes

CHAPTER 7

PUTTING IT ALL TOGETHER: MEAL PLANNING AND MORE

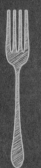

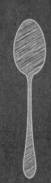

I used to think meal planning was for extremely organized people. It turns out, meal planning is a necessity when you are a little less than organized, short on time, and low on budget.

In my case, I'd go nuts without having a master plan for my family. Working full-time and juggling three kids and all their activities leaves very little time to do anything on the fly.

It wasn't until my children went to school that I began to incorporate lunches into my weekly plan. I began to see the benefits of meal planning shortly after I began planning our dinners and writing out a grocery list. Lunches however, were often forgotten, or I'd run out of ingredients.

For this reason, I now teach thousands of parents how to incorporate lunches into the dinner plan over at MOMables.com. Lunch is, after all, one-third of what we eat each day!

Meal Planning 101

Following are some of my best weekly meal planning tips and techniques. They should get you started with ease!

- Create a master list of meals that includes healthy and quick homemade dinners your family loves. Whether you bookmark them on the Internet or print them out and store them in a binder, keep them all in one place.

- Write down what you will make for lunch for the week. Try out new recipes from this book as well as old favorites, and check out the ingredients you'll need.

- Look at your planned lunches, and see if you can create shortcuts for yourself while you are making dinner. I've made sure to include lots of plan-ahead tips in most of the recipes.

- Schedule a prep day. Set aside some time to prep foods that will be healthy grab-and-go options for lunch and snacks.

- Bake treats and breakfast items while you are cooking dinner or right after, when your kitchen is more likely to be dirty and the oven already on.

- Remember your leftovers! Check the contents of your fridge, and put one of the awesome recipes in this book to use.

- Wash all produce (except raspberries) as soon as you get home from the grocery.

- Think of your crockpot as your kitchen assistant when you are off-duty.

- Get the kids involved in selecting the recipes they would like to try!

Sample Meal Plans

Here's what a sample meal plan might look like in my house. Charts go a long way in keeping me on track!

WEEK 1	Breakfast	Lunch
Monday	Kitchen Sink Muffins (page 35), fresh berries	Veggie Skewers (page 119), hummus, The Frenchman (page 53)
Tuesday	Eggs-to-Go (page 36)	Ninja Turtle Grilled Cheese (page 57), sliced apples
Wednesday	Kitchen Sink Muffins (page 35)	Chicken Cordon Bleu Pasta (page 145), Banana Split Bites (page 210)
Thursday	Build Your Own Parfait (page 125), granola	Homemade O's (page 145), Rainbow Fruit Cups (page 202)
Friday	Eggs-to-Go (page 36)	Grilled Chicken, Cheddar, grapes, carrots, Greek Yogurt Dip (page 177)

WEEK 2	Breakfast	Lunch
Monday	1 cup (230 g) yogurt, ¼ cup (112 g) granola, berries	Pesto Lover's Box (page 132), Parmesan Crostinis (page 169), Rainbow Fruit Cups (page 202)
Tuesday	Cinnamon Roll Overnight Oatmeal (page 40)	Mashed Chickpea Sandwich (page 79), Flourless Chocolate Cookies (page 211), orange slices
Wednesday	Breakfast Burrito (page 36)	Neighborhood Meatballs (page 104), Parmesan Crostinis (page 169), Rainbow Fruit Cups (page 202)
Thursday	Blueberry Bread (page 163), ½ cup (125 g) sliced peaches	Grilled Taco Sandwich (page 46), sliced apples, Homemade Salsa (page 180)
Friday	Orange Push-Pop Smoothie (page 189)	ABC Pinwheels (page 89), salsa, Caramel Banilla Bites (page 202)

WEEK 1	Snack	Dinner
Monday	Peaches and Cream Smoothie (page 190)	Chicken Cordon Bleu Pasta (page 145), salad
Tuesday	Ladybugs (page 196)	Homemade O's (page 145), salad
Wednesday	Greek Yogurt Dip (page 177), carrots	Grilled chicken, steamed broccoli, Bombay Rice (page 138)
Thursday	Kettle Corn (page 201)	Ginger Carrots (page 155), dumplings, salad
Friday	Mango Madness Smoothie (page 181)	Family Pizza Night: Pizza Dough (page 167), salad

WEEK 2	Snack	Dinner
Monday	Frozen Yogurt Berries (page 205)	Breakfast Night: Whole Wheat Waffles (page 44), scrambled eggs, fruit
Tuesday	White Chocolate Peanut Butter and Strawberry Crostinis (page 208)	Taco Night: ground beef, soft tortillas, shredded cheese, Homemade Salsa (page 180), Easy Guacamole (page 180), sour cream, black beans
Wednesday	Peaches and Cream Smoothie (page 190)	Neighborhood Meatballs (page 104), spaghetti, salad
Thursday	The Hulk (Green Smoothie) (page 181)	Creamy Avocado Pasta (page 141), salad
Friday	Sweet Ants on a Log (page 198)	Tuna Quinoa Casserole (page 137), salad

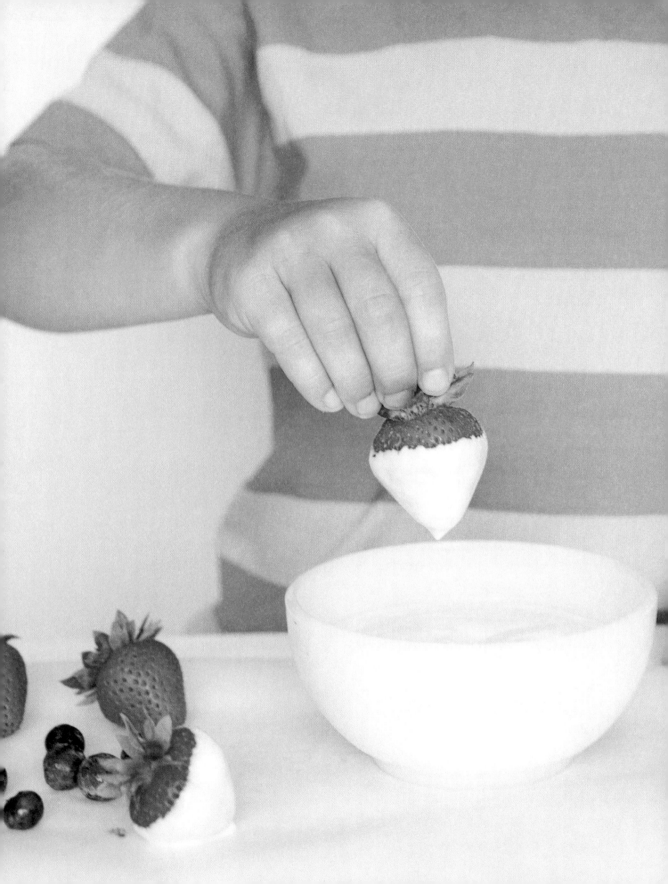

Healthy Snacks on the Go

As a busy mom with kids in after-school activities, I often feel like a chauffeur who lives in her minivan.

So what happens when the kids start getting hungry between shuttle stops? They get cranky, and if this momma doesn't have snacks packed, things turn into the "van of doom," since I refuse to buy junk at a drive-through.

Here are my go-to snacks and how to pack them for minimal van cleanup:

- Strawberry Fruit Leather (page 84); bring wet wipes for sticky hands
- Blueberry Bread slices (page 163) in small individual containers
- Cheese sticks rolled inside ham slices
- Carrot and celery sticks with Homemade Ranch Dressing Mix (page 175) in a dipper container
- White Bean Dip (page 177) with veggies or crackers in a divided container
- Peanut Butter Fruit Dip (page 179) with apple slices
- Ladybugs (page 196), deconstructed in a divided container
- Maple Glazed Trail Mix (page 198)
- Oatmeal Raisin Granola Bar (page 206) and fresh strawberries in a divided container
- Smoothies in a jar (keep frozen for long road trips, and they'll thaw during the drive)

Classroom Snacks

The year my daughter entered preschool, I learned how challenging it was to bring snacks for an entire classroom of toddlers once every two weeks. When I asked the teachers what I should bring, they told me to just buy cookies and crackers in individual bags. Not my style!

Below is my list of go-to healthy alternatives to store-bought and how I pack them in individual portions for each student. (Don't forget to make a few extra bags just in case!)

- Kitchen Sink Muffins (page 35), packaged in ziplock sandwich bags

- Breakfast Cookies (page 38), packaged in ziplock sandwich bags

- One small apple plus individual string cheese stick (if you freeze string cheese, it will thaw and be cold by snack time)

- Lunchbox Cheese Crackers (page 192), packaged in snack-size ziplock bags

- Protein Cookie Bites (page 194) made with sunflower seed butter (to avoid possible allergy), packaged in snack-size ziplock bags (two cookie bites per bag)

- Maple Glazed Trail Mix (page 198) or Kettle Corn (page 201), packaged in ziplock sandwich bags

- Rainbow Fruit Cups (page 202), packaged in small disposable containers

- Oatmeal Raisin Granola Bars (page 206), packaged in snack-size ziplock bags

- Gallon-size jug filled with any of the smoothie recipes in this book, sent with disposable kid-size cups

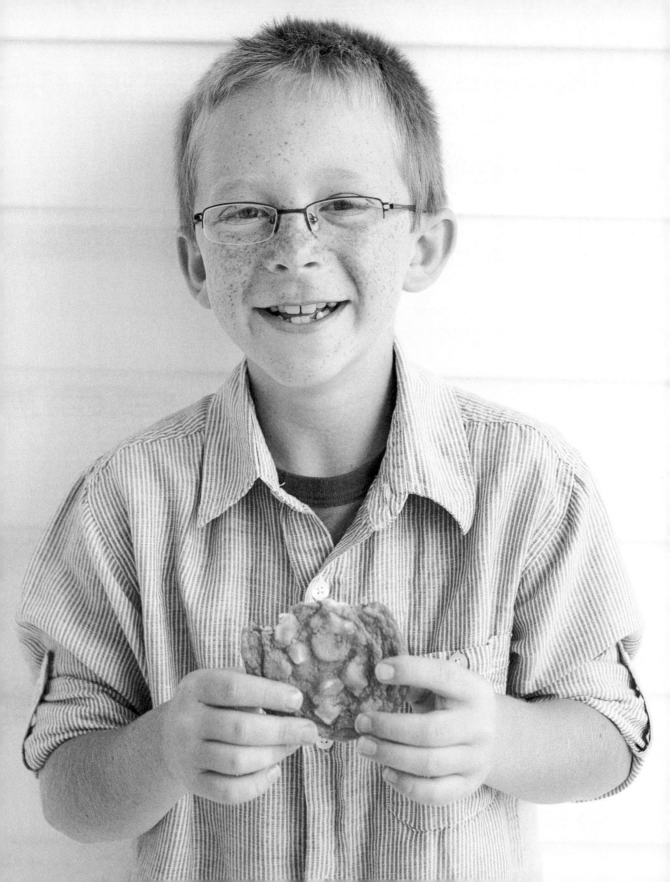

Feedback Chart

Use this section as a guide to track all the delicious dishes you've created from this book. Let the kids fill in the star ratings so it's quick and easy to go back and find their favorites!

RECIPE	DATE MADE	KID STAR RATING (Fill in the stars!)	NOTES (Any recipe adjustments or variations made? Was this served with other items? Recipe good for make-ahead?)	MAKE AGAIN?
GET OUT THE DOOR: BREAKFASTS TO GO				
Perfect Pancakes (page 33)		☆☆☆☆☆		◯ YES ◯ NO
Kitchen Sink Muffins (page 35)		☆☆☆☆☆		◯ YES ◯ NO
Eggs-to-Go (page 36)		☆☆☆☆☆		◯ YES ◯ NO
Breakfast Burrito (page 36)		☆☆☆☆☆		◯ YES ◯ NO
Breakfast Cookies (page 38)		☆☆☆☆☆		◯ YES ◯ NO
French Toast Stix (page 40)		☆☆☆☆☆		◯ YES ◯ NO
Cinnamon Roll Overnight Oatmeal (page 40)		☆☆☆☆☆		◯ YES ◯ NO
Chocolate Chip Freezer Scones (page 41)		☆☆☆☆☆		◯ YES ◯ NO
Glazed Cake Donut Muffins (page 43)		☆☆☆☆☆		◯ YES ◯ NO
Lunchbox Granola (page 44)		☆☆☆☆☆		◯ YES ◯ NO
Whole Wheat Waffles (page 44)		☆☆☆☆☆		◯ YES ◯ NO
FILL THE BOX: SANDWICHES AND MORE				
Avocado Bacon Melt (page 46)		☆☆☆☆☆		◯ YES ◯ NO
Grilled Taco Sandwich (page 46)		☆☆☆☆☆		◯ YES ◯ NO
Pretzelwich (page 47)		☆☆☆☆☆		◯ YES ◯ NO

RECIPE	DATE MADE	KID STAR RATING	NOTES	MAKE AGAIN?
Egg Salad Sandwich (page 47)		☆☆☆☆☆		○ YES ○ NO
Angel Food Sandwich (page 49)		☆☆☆☆☆		○ YES ○ NO
Candy Apple Sandwich (page 49)		☆☆☆☆☆		○ YES ○ NO
Ricotta and Jam Pancake Sandwich (page 51)		☆☆☆☆☆		○ YES ○ NO
Honey Bee Sandwich (page 51)		☆☆☆☆☆		○ YES ○ NO
Hummus Avocado Sandwich (page 52)		☆☆☆☆☆		○ YES ○ NO
Grilled Harvest Sandwich (page 52)		☆☆☆☆☆		○ YES ○ NO
The Frenchman (page 53)		☆☆☆☆☆		○ YES ○ NO
Boy Meets Girl Sandwich (page 53)		☆☆☆☆☆		○ YES ○ NO
Grilled Chicken and Pesto Sandwich (page 55)		☆☆☆☆☆		○ YES ○ NO
Barbecue Chicken Sandwich (page 55)		☆☆☆☆☆		○ YES ○ NO
Grilled Chicken, Cheddar, and Grapes (page 56)		☆☆☆☆☆		○ YES ○ NO
Ricotta and Pesto Sandwich (page 56)		☆☆☆☆☆		○ YES ○ NO
Ninja Turtle Grilled Cheese (page 57)		☆☆☆☆☆		○ YES ○ NO
Grilled Leprechaun (page 57)		☆☆☆☆☆		○ YES ○ NO
Veggie Club (page 59)		☆☆☆☆☆		○ YES ○ NO
Turkey and Hummus Sandwich (page 59)		☆☆☆☆☆		○ YES ○ NO
Apple Pie Sandwiches (page 60)		☆☆☆☆☆		○ YES ○ NO
Blueberry Heaven (page 60)		☆☆☆☆☆		○ YES ○ NO
Sunny Side Sandwich (page 62)		☆☆☆☆☆		○ YES ○ NO

RECIPE	DATE MADE	KID STAR RATING	NOTES	MAKE AGAIN?
Peaches and Cream Wafflewich (page 62)		☆☆☆☆☆		○ YES ○ NO
Strawberry Grilled Cheese (page 64)		☆☆☆☆☆		○ YES ○ NO
Strawberry Kiwi Wafflewich (page 64)		☆☆☆☆☆		○ YES ○ NO
Lemon Sorbet Sandwich (page 66)		☆☆☆☆☆		○ YES ○ NO
Dreamsicle Sandwich (page 66)		☆☆☆☆☆		○ YES ○ NO
Berrylicious Sandwich (page 67)		☆☆☆☆☆		○ YES ○ NO
Roast Beef Farmer's Sandwich (page 67)		☆☆☆☆☆		○ YES ○ NO
Kid's Philly Steak Sandwich (page 68)		☆☆☆☆☆		○ YES ○ NO
Easy Muffuletta (page 68)		☆☆☆☆☆		○ YES ○ NO
California Turkey Avocado Sandwich (page 70)		☆☆☆☆☆		○ YES ○ NO
Grilled Meat Loaf Sandwich (page 70)		☆☆☆☆☆		○ YES ○ NO
Skinny Elvis (page 71)		☆☆☆☆☆		○ YES ○ NO
The Elephant Sandwich (page 71)		☆☆☆☆☆		○ YES ○ NO
Grilled Italian (page 73)		☆☆☆☆☆		○ YES ○ NO
Swiss Tuna Melt (page 73)		☆☆☆☆☆		○ YES ○ NO
Avocado Delight (page 75)		☆☆☆☆☆		○ YES ○ NO
Hummus Monster (page 75)		☆☆☆☆☆		○ YES ○ NO
The Nathan (page 77)		☆☆☆☆☆		○ YES ○ NO
Ham and Cheese "Waffle" (page 77)		☆☆☆☆☆		○ YES ○ NO
Mashed Chickpea Sandwich (page 79)		☆☆☆☆☆		○ YES ○ NO
Pure Pastrami (page 80)		☆☆☆☆☆		○ YES ○ NO

RECIPE	DATE MADE	KID STAR RATING	NOTES	MAKE AGAIN?
Hawaiian Sliders (page 80)		☆☆☆☆☆		○ YES ○ NO
Chicken Salad Sliders (page 82)		☆☆☆☆☆		○ YES ○ NO
Cucumber Goat Cheese Sliders (page 82)		☆☆☆☆☆		○ YES ○ NO
Caprese Sliders (page 83)		☆☆☆☆☆		○ YES ○ NO
Norwegian Tea Sandwich (page 83)		☆☆☆☆☆		○ YES ○ NO
PB & J Pinwheels (page 84)		☆☆☆☆☆		○ YES ○ NO
Strawberry Fruit Leather (page 84)		☆☆☆☆☆		○ YES ○ NO
Hawaiian Puff-Wheels (page 87)		☆☆☆☆☆		○ YES ○ NO
Cuban Pinwheels (page 87)		☆☆☆☆☆		○ YES ○ NO
ABC Pinwheels (page 89)		☆☆☆☆☆		○ YES ○ NO
Tapenade Pinwheels (page 89)		☆☆☆☆☆		○ YES ○ NO
Pesto Swirls (page 90)		☆☆☆☆☆		○ YES ○ NO
Chocolate Flautas (page 91)		☆☆☆☆☆		○ YES ○ NO
Honey Mustard Chicken Wrap (page 91)		☆☆☆☆☆		○ YES ○ NO
Crunchy Carrot Wrap (page 92)		☆☆☆☆☆		○ YES ○ NO
All My Veggies Wrap (page 92)		☆☆☆☆☆		○ YES ○ NO
Little Italy Wrap (page 92)		☆☆☆☆☆		○ YES ○ NO
Turkey Avocado Wrap (page 92)		☆☆☆☆☆		○ YES ○ NO
Pizza Man Wheels (page 93)		☆☆☆☆☆		○ YES ○ NO
Black Bean Quesadillas (page 95)		☆☆☆☆☆		○ YES ○ NO
Pizza Dough Stromboli (page 96)		☆☆☆☆☆		○ YES ○ NO

RECIPE	DATE MADE	KID STAR RATING	NOTES	MAKE AGAIN?
Pizza Dippers (page 97)		☆☆☆☆☆		○ YES ○ NO
Green Eggs and Ham Pizza (page 97)		☆☆☆☆☆		○ YES ○ NO
Cheddar and Pear Quesadillas (page 99)		☆☆☆☆☆		○ YES ○ NO
Baked Raviolis (page 101)		☆☆☆☆☆		○ YES ○ NO
Pesto Pasta (page 102)		☆☆☆☆☆		○ YES ○ NO
Garden Fresh Pasta (page 102)		☆☆☆☆☆		○ YES ○ NO
Italian Pasta Salad (page 103)		☆☆☆☆☆		○ YES ○ NO
Greek Orzo Pasta Salad (page 103)		☆☆☆☆☆		○ YES ○ NO
Neighborhood Meatballs (page 104)		☆☆☆☆☆		○ YES ○ NO
Meatball Dippers (page 105)		☆☆☆☆☆		○ YES ○ NO
Olives and Feta Lego Pasta (page 106)		☆☆☆☆☆		○ YES ○ NO
Arriba! Seasoning (page 106)		☆☆☆☆☆		○ YES ○ NO
Arriba! Pasta Salad (page 107)		☆☆☆☆☆		○ YES ○ NO
Southern Chicken Salad (page 108)		☆☆☆☆☆		○ YES ○ NO
Dad's Tuna Pasta Salad (page 108)		☆☆☆☆☆		○ YES ○ NO
Mexican Pasta Salad (page 109)		☆☆☆☆☆		○ YES ○ NO
Avocado Tuna Salad (page 109)		☆☆☆☆☆		○ YES ○ NO
No Mayo Egg Salad (page 110)		☆☆☆☆☆		○ YES ○ NO
Big Jim's Chicken Salad (page 110)		☆☆☆☆☆		○ YES ○ NO
Veggie Meat Loaf (page 111)		☆☆☆☆☆		○ YES ○ NO
Grilled Cheese Dippers (page 113)		☆☆☆☆☆		○ YES ○ NO

RECIPE	DATE MADE	KID STAR RATING	NOTES	MAKE AGAIN?
Spaghetti Tacos (page 113)		☆☆☆☆☆		○ YES ○ NO
Lunchbox Falafels (page 115)		☆☆☆☆☆		○ YES ○ NO
Olive Strips (page 115)		☆☆☆☆☆		○ YES ○ NO
Easy Peasy Frittata (page 116)		☆☆☆☆☆		○ YES ○ NO
ADD SOME FUN: INTERACTIVE LUNCHES FOR PICKY EATERS				
Tortellini Swords (page 119)		☆☆☆☆☆		○ YES ○ NO
Veggie Skewers (page 119)		☆☆☆☆☆		○ YES ○ NO
Real Chicken Nuggets (page 120)		☆☆☆☆☆		○ YES ○ NO
Spaghetti Cupcakes (page 121)		☆☆☆☆☆		○ YES ○ NO
Build Your Own Pizza Lunch (page 121)		☆☆☆☆☆		○ YES ○ NO
Ham and Cheese Swords (page 123)		☆☆☆☆☆		○ YES ○ NO
Build Your Own Roman Army Boats (page 123)		☆☆☆☆☆		○ YES ○ NO
Mini Quiches (page 125)		☆☆☆☆☆		○ YES ○ NO
Build Your Own Parfait (page 125)		☆☆☆☆☆		○ YES ○ NO
Mac and Cheese Bites (page 126)		☆☆☆☆☆		○ YES ○ NO
Monkey Towers (page 126)		☆☆☆☆☆		○ YES ○ NO
Veggie Nuggets (page 127)		☆☆☆☆☆		○ YES ○ NO
The Original MOMable (page 129)		☆☆☆☆☆		○ YES ○ NO
Old School Cracker Stackers (page 129)		☆☆☆☆☆		○ YES ○ NO
Peach Cobbler Box (page 131)		☆☆☆☆☆		○ YES ○ NO
Monkey Hot Dog (page 131)		☆☆☆☆☆		○ YES ○ NO

RECIPE	DATE MADE	KID STAR RATING	NOTES	MAKE AGAIN?
Quinoa Bites (page 132)		☆☆☆☆☆		○ YES ○ NO
Pesto Lover's Box (page 132)		☆☆☆☆☆		○ YES ○ NO
Baked Mozzarella Sticks (page 134)		☆☆☆☆☆		○ YES ○ NO
Baked Zucchini Fries (page 135)		☆☆☆☆☆		○ YES ○ NO
FILL THE THERMOS: PORTABLE HOT LUNCHES				
Tuna Quinoa Casserole (page 137)		☆☆☆☆☆		○ YES ○ NO
Dad's Fried Rice (page 138)		☆☆☆☆☆		○ YES ○ NO
Bombay Rice (page 138)		☆☆☆☆☆		○ YES ○ NO
Stoplight Rice (page 140)		☆☆☆☆☆		○ YES ○ NO
Bacon, Corn, and Avocado Macaroni (page 140)		☆☆☆☆☆		○ YES ○ NO
Creamy Avocado Pasta (page 141)		☆☆☆☆☆		○ YES ○ NO
Peasy Tortellini (page 141)		☆☆☆☆☆		○ YES ○ NO
Margarita Pasta Salad (page 143)		☆☆☆☆☆		○ YES ○ NO
Homemade Alfredo Sauce (page 143)		☆☆☆☆☆		○ YES ○ NO
Veggie Tomato Sauce (page 144)		☆☆☆☆☆		○ YES ○ NO
Homemade O's (page 145)		☆☆☆☆☆		○ YES ○ NO
Chicken Cordon Bleu Pasta (page 145)		☆☆☆☆☆		○ YES ○ NO
Midweek Penne Bake (page 146)		☆☆☆☆☆		○ YES ○ NO
Broccoroni (page 146)		☆☆☆☆☆		○ YES ○ NO
No Cheese Mac 'n Cheese (page 147)		☆☆☆☆☆		○ YES ○ NO
Zucchini Pasta (page 147)		☆☆☆☆☆		○ YES ○ NO

RECIPE	DATE MADE	KID STAR RATING	NOTES	MAKE AGAIN?
Red Beans and Rice (page 149)		☆☆☆☆☆		○ YES ○ NO
Dad's Easy Bean Soup (page 149)		☆☆☆☆☆		○ YES ○ NO
Tomato Veggie Soup (page 150)		☆☆☆☆☆		○ YES ○ NO
White Bean Pumpkin Soup (page 150)		☆☆☆☆☆		○ YES ○ NO
Homemade Ramen (page 151)		☆☆☆☆☆		○ YES ○ NO
Chicken Taco Soup (page 151)		☆☆☆☆☆		○ YES ○ NO
Mexican Soup (page 153)		☆☆☆☆☆		○ YES ○ NO
Tortellini Soup (page 153)		☆☆☆☆☆		○ YES ○ NO
Lasagna Soup (page 154)		☆☆☆☆☆		○ YES ○ NO
Lentil Soup (page 155)		☆☆☆☆☆		○ YES ○ NO
Ginger Carrots (page 155)		☆☆☆☆☆		○ YES ○ NO
Southwest Quinoa (page 157)		☆☆☆☆☆		○ YES ○ NO
Lunchbox Baked Potato (page 158)		☆☆☆☆☆		○ YES ○ NO
Dumplings Lunch (page 158)		☆☆☆☆☆		○ YES ○ NO
Mini Tuna Balls (page 159)		☆☆☆☆☆		○ YES ○ NO
Chicken Teriyaki Bowl (page 159)		☆☆☆☆☆		○ YES ○ NO

EXTRA CREDIT: STAPLES, DRINKS, TREATS, AND MORE

RECIPE	DATE MADE	KID STAR RATING	NOTES	MAKE AGAIN?
Honey Wheat Biscuits (page 161)		☆☆☆☆☆		○ YES ○ NO
Blueberry Bread (page 163)		☆☆☆☆☆		○ YES ○ NO
Lemon Bread (page 164)		☆☆☆☆☆		○ YES ○ NO
Peanut Butter Bread (page 164)		☆☆☆☆☆		○ YES ○ NO

RECIPE	DATE MADE	KID STAR RATING	NOTES	MAKE AGAIN?
Banana Bread (page 165)		☆☆☆☆☆		○ YES ○ NO
Pizza Dough (page 167)		☆☆☆☆☆		○ YES ○ NO
Cornbread Muffins (page 169)		☆☆☆☆☆		○ YES ○ NO
Parmesan Crostinis (page 169)		☆☆☆☆☆		○ YES ○ NO
Easy Freezer Jam (page 170)		☆☆☆☆☆		○ YES ○ NO
Cinnamon Raisin Peanut Butter (page 170)		☆☆☆☆☆		○ YES ○ NO
Easy Homemade Chocolate Spread (page 171)		☆☆☆☆☆		○ YES ○ NO
Caramel Peanut Butter (page 171)		☆☆☆☆☆		○ YES ○ NO
White Chocolate Peanut Butter (page 173)		☆☆☆☆☆		○ YES ○ NO
Flavored Cream Cheese (page 173)		☆☆☆☆☆		○ YES ○ NO
Homemade Pesto (page 174)		☆☆☆☆☆		○ YES ○ NO
Olive Salad (page 174)		☆☆☆☆☆		○ YES ○ NO
Homemade Ranch Dressing Mix (page 175)		☆☆☆☆☆		○ YES ○ NO
Greek Hummus (page 175)		☆☆☆☆☆		○ YES ○ NO
White Bean Dip (page 177)		☆☆☆☆☆		○ YES ○ NO
Greek Yogurt Dip (page 177)		☆☆☆☆☆		○ YES ○ NO
Peanut Butter Fruit Dip (page 179)		☆☆☆☆☆		○ YES ○ NO
Cinnamon Crunch Dip (page 179)		☆☆☆☆☆		○ YES ○ NO
Cookie Dough Dip (page 179)		☆☆☆☆☆		○ YES ○ NO
Easy Guacamole (page 180)		☆☆☆☆☆		○ YES ○ NO

RECIPE	DATE MADE	KID STAR RATING	NOTES	MAKE AGAIN?
Homemade Salsa (page 180)		☆☆☆☆☆		○ YES ○ NO
Mango Madness Smoothie (page 181)		☆☆☆☆☆		○ YES ○ NO
The Hulk (Green Smoothie) (page 181)		☆☆☆☆☆		○ YES ○ NO
Blueberry Lemonade Smoothie (page 185)		☆☆☆☆☆		○ YES ○ NO
Coconut Pie Smoothie (page 185)		☆☆☆☆☆		○ YES ○ NO
Chocolate Chip Cookie Smoothie (page 186)		☆☆☆☆☆		○ YES ○ NO
Homemade Chocolate Syrup (page 186)		☆☆☆☆☆		○ YES ○ NO
Peanut Butter Cup Smoothie (page 188)		☆☆☆☆☆		○ YES ○ NO
Big Athlete Shake (page 188)		☆☆☆☆☆		○ YES ○ NO
Orange Push-Pop Smoothie (page 189)		☆☆☆☆☆		○ YES ○ NO
Bugs Bunny Smoothie (page 189)		☆☆☆☆☆		○ YES ○ NO
Vitamin C Cubes (page 190)		☆☆☆☆☆		○ YES ○ NO
Peaches and Cream Smoothie (page 190)		☆☆☆☆☆		○ YES ○ NO
Lunchbox Cheese Crackers (page 192)		☆☆☆☆☆		○ YES ○ NO
Protein Cookie Bites (page 194)		☆☆☆☆☆		○ YES ○ NO
Chocolate Athlete Bars (page 195)		☆☆☆☆☆		○ YES ○ NO
Chocolate Chip Date Bars (page 196)		☆☆☆☆☆		○ YES ○ NO
Ladybugs (page 196)		☆☆☆☆☆		○ YES ○ NO
Sweet Ants on a Log (page 198)		☆☆☆☆☆		○ YES ○ NO
Maple Glazed Trail Mix (page 198)		☆☆☆☆☆		○ YES ○ NO
Cinnamon Raisin Newtons (page 199)		☆☆☆☆☆		○ YES ○ NO

RECIPE	DATE MADE	KID STAR RATING	NOTES	MAKE AGAIN?
Kettle Corn (page 201)		☆☆☆☆☆		○ YES ○ NO
Caramel Banilla Bites (page 202)		☆☆☆☆☆		○ YES ○ NO
Rainbow Fruit Cups (page 202)		☆☆☆☆☆		○ YES ○ NO
Frozen Yogurt Berries (page 205)		☆☆☆☆☆		○ YES ○ NO
No-Bake Brownie Bites (page 205)		☆☆☆☆☆		○ YES ○ NO
Oatmeal Raisin Granola Bars (page 206)		☆☆☆☆☆		○ YES ○ NO
Strawberry Shortcake Kabobs (page 208)		☆☆☆☆☆		○ YES ○ NO
White Chocolate Peanut Butter Strawberry Crostinis (page 208)		☆☆☆☆☆		○ YES ○ NO
Banana Split Bites (page 210)		☆☆☆☆☆		○ YES ○ NO
Flourless Chocolate Cookies (page 211)		☆☆☆☆☆		○ YES ○ NO
Halloween Loot Cookies (page 212)		☆☆☆☆☆		○ YES ○ NO
White Chocolate Chip Cookies (page 212)		☆☆☆☆☆		○ YES ○ NO
Classroom Cupcakes (page 215)		☆☆☆☆☆		○ YES ○ NO

Acknowledgments

To Eric, my best friend and love of my life. Without your support and encouragement, this cookbook would not have come to fruition. Thank you for reminding me that I can achieve greatness and that I am enough.

To my kids, Sofia, Alex, and Gabriel. Thank you for being a challenge to cook for. Little did I know that trying to feed you better would help thousands along the way. You are my inspiration, my gift, and my life's work.

To my parents, John and Isabel. I am forever grateful for helping me launch my business, believing in me when I didn't, and for encouraging my creativity in the world of lunch. I love that you've known I could do *anything* all along.

To my in-laws, Moose and Debbie. For possibly the best summer my kids will ever have, filled with love, activities, and fun over at grammie camp. Without your help, I could not have tested recipes, worked every weekend for nearly four months, and written this book.

To my MOMables team. Thank you for going along with whatever recipe I've sent your way. For helping me grow my dream and inspiring thousands. You are amazing.

To my friend, Alison Bickel. You've been so giving, trusting, and an amazing photography teacher. I love that you can photograph my recipes better than I could ever explain. I can't imagine doing a cookbook without you.

To the thousands of lunch packers in the MOMables community. You inspire me and make me want to work harder to find ways to help you feed your kids fresh lunches.

To Amanda, my editor. Your guidance and help has been instrumental to this cookbook-writing rookie.

To my friend, Kelly. For your support, love, and tirelessly giving of your time. I am grateful for your editing and unconditional love.

To our Creator. With you, all things are possible.

About the Author

Laura Fuentes is the founder and CEO of MOMables.com, where she helps thousands of parents every day make lunches their kids will love.

Laura is a speaker, recipe developer, and lover of all things mom. She partners with major real food brands to promote healthy school lunches, reduce childhood obesity, and teach healthy family eating.

In her personal blog, Laura writes about motherhood, good family food, managing deadlines, and keeping her cool, even when her kids super-glued her hair.

Above all, her most important job is caring for her family.

To find out more about Laura, visit www.LauraFuentes.com.

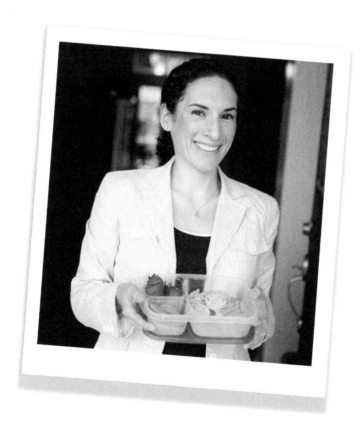

Index